Heart Smart

A Cardiologist's 5-Step Plan for
Detecting, Preventing, and
Even Reversing Heart Disease

Matthew S. DeVane, D.O., F.A.C.C.

WILEY

John Wiley & Sons, Inc.

Published by John Wiley & Sons, Inc., Hoboken, New Jersey
Published simultaneously in Canada

Design and composition by Navta Associates, Inc.

Limit of Liability/Disclaimer of Warranty: The information contained in this book is not intended to serve as a replacement for professional medical advice. Any use of the information in this book is at the reader's discretion. The author and the publisher specifically disclaim any and all liability arising directly or indirectly from the use or application of any information contained in this book. A health care professional should be consulted regarding your specific situation.

For general information about our other products and services, please contact our Customer Care Department within the United States at (800) 762-2974, outside the United States at (317) 572-3993 or fax (317) 572-4002.

Wiley also publishes its books in a variety of electronic formats. Some content that appears in print may not be available in electronic books. For more information about Wiley products, visit our web site at www.wiley.com.

Library of Congress Cataloging-in-Publication Data:
DeVane, Matthew S., date
    Heart smart : a cardiologist's 5-step plan for detecting, preventing, and even reversing heart disease / Matthew S. DeVane.
        p. cm.
    ISBN-13 978-0-471-74692-8 (cloth)
    ISBN-10 0-471-74692-4 (cloth)
1. Heart—Diseases—Popular works. 2. Heart—Diseases—Diagnosis—Popular works. 3. Heart—Diseases—Prevention—Popular works. 4. Heart—Diseases—Risk factors—Popular works. I. Title.
    RC672.D48 2006
    616.1'2—dc22   2005031917

Printed in the United States of America

10 9 8 7 6 5 4 3 2 1

In loving memory of my father,
Ernest William DeVane Jr.

Contents

Foreword

Heart disease kills more men and women in the United States every year than any other disease. In fact, over 41 percent of all deaths in the United States each year result from heart disease. If you combine heart disease and stroke, the two major vascular diseases, these two entities kill more men and women in the United States every year than all diseases combined!

Consider the following facts:

- One American dies of heart disease every 33 seconds—almost one million deaths every year.

- Almost 25 percent of adults in the United States have one or more types of heart disease.

- If you consider all risk factors for heart disease such as elevated cholesterol, cigarette smoking, high blood pressure, physical inactivity, and being overweight or obese, there isn't a single family in America left untouched by heart disease.

With these grim statistics in mind, it is imperative that we in the cardiology community make every effort to educate our patients about heart disease and what they can do about it. In this important new book, *Heart Smart: A Cardiologist's 5-Step Plan for Detecting, Preventing, and Even Reversing Heart Disease*, Dr. Matthew DeVane has done just that.

Dr. DeVane combines the latest information on all aspects of heart disease with a user-friendly, motivational writing style, which will certainly help individuals lower their risk of ever developing heart disease or more effectively manage it if they currently have one of the forms of heart disease or other vascular conditions.

A great strength of this book is Dr. DeVane's clear and lucid explanation of risk factors and what each individual can do to lower the chance of ever developing heart disease. It is critically important that we emphasize to our patients how much power they have in their own hands to lower their risk of heart disease. Let me give you an example. A study published recently in the prestigious *New England Journal of Medicine* showed that over 80 pecent of all heart disease in women could be eliminated if individuals would take the following actions:

- Stop smoking
- Increase physical activity
- Improve nutritional habits
- Maintain a proper body weight

Despite these very encouraging predictions, only 3 percent of women in this study met all four of these criteria. We need to do a better job!

Another great strength of Dr. DeVane's book is the clear explanation of current and emerging technologies, which assist us in the early detection of various forms of heart disease. Such emerging technologies as cardiac MRI and high-speed CT of the coronary arteries provide early information that was never accessible to cardiologists before. Dr. DeVane describes each of these and many other tests in detail and offers sound advice about who should have each test and what information each test yields.

I believe that the greatest opportunity to lower the tremendous toll of heart disease in the United States is to convince our patients that the best results come from a partnership between them and their doctor. Dr. DeVane's authoritative guide will provide tremendous help in this educational process.

This is an important book addressing key health considerations relevant to every family in America. I urge every adult to read *Heart Smart* and every cardiologist's office to stock it and recommend it to their patients.

It is through efforts such as Dr. DeVane's work that we will finally begin to make inroads into the enormous problem of cardiovascular disease in the United States.

James M. Rippe, M.D.
Associate Professor of Medicine
   (Cardiology), Tufts University School
   of Medicine
Founder and Director, Rippe Lifestyle
   Institute and Rippe Health Assessment

Acknowledgments

Thanks to Hector Fontanet, M.D., my mentor, and all my friends at the Florida Cardiovascular Institute in Tampa, Florida. Thanks to my agent, Carol Susan Roth, at the Carol Susan Roth Literary Agency. It is safe to say that without Carol there would be no *Heart Smart*. Carol's wisdom, aggressiveness, and determination turned my ideas into a proposal and my proposal into a book. Carol also introduced me to another Carol—Carol Whitely, who provided expert editing, proofreading, and emotional support.

Many thanks to the best cardiology group in the country—my friends and partners at Cardiovascular Consultants Medical Group in the East Bay of northern California. Thanks to Thomas Miller and Teryn Kendall at John Wiley & Sons for believing in me and making my dream a reality.

Special thanks go out to my patients. It is an honor and the highest privilege to be your cardiologist. I look forward to a happy and *healthy* relationship for years and years to come. Lastly, thanks to my wife, Barb, and my three sweet angels—Emily, Abby, and Allison.

Introduction

The Heart Smart Advantage

Bill had worked hard to get his weight back down to where it should be. He was exercising regularly, had good blood pressure, and was managing to suppress and control his weakness for fast food. He was an influential and powerful man of fifty-eight who had regular checkups and testing with the best doctors and the best hospitals in the world.

Dave, like Bill, seemed to be the picture of good health. Dave wasn't overweight; indeed, he looked to be a little on the thin side. At fifty-two he worked hard and had access to and the means to get the best health care that money could buy.

Yet somehow these two healthy-seeming baby boomers ended up with severe coronary heart disease that went completely undetected until they both needed urgent open-heart bypass surgery.

Who were Bill and Dave? I'm talking about President Bill Clinton and Late Show *host David Letterman.*

When you read about the heart-health problems of these very prominent men, you might think that if a president and a celebrity television host, with all they have access to, couldn't detect their heart disease early, then what chance do I have of finding it early enough to prevent serious heart issues? Well, you do have a chance, and I guarantee that by reading *Heart Smart* and taking advantage of new technology and available tests, you can detect heart disease early and have the best opportunity to avoid bypass surgery or perhaps even a heart attack.

The Heart Smart Advantage

Heart Smart is a must read for anyone interested in heart disease prevention. Unlike all the other heart-health books available on the market, *Heart Smart*:

1

- Is authored by a cardiologist specializing in and dedicated to heart disease prevention.
- Tells you how to utilize traditional cardiac risk factors, emerging cardiac risk factors, and state-of-the-art technology to help you defeat coronary heart disease.
- Provides a proven, successful strategy of exercise, nutrition, heart-healthy superfoods, and supplements as well as medications to lower your cardiac risk and prevent heart attacks.

Well-Known Baby Boomers Who Had Cardiovascular Disease

Former president Bill Clinton: four-vessel bypass surgery (age fifty-eight)

John Ritter (actor): died from a tear in his aorta (age fifty-four)

David Letterman (Late Show TV host): five-vessel bypass surgery (age fifty-two)

Dana Carvey (actor/comedian): two-vessel bypass surgery (age forty-two)

Robert Palmer (recording artist): sudden cardiac death (age fifty-four)

Jim Cantalupo (CEO of McDonald's): sudden cardiac death (age sixty)

How to Use This Book

As a cardiologist in private practice who works every day on the "front lines," I have used my clinical experience along with up-to-date clinical data and national guidelines to develop a comprehensive, proven, and effective five-step program for heart disease prevention. My program is easy to understand, and once you start it I know you'll be on your way to better heart health.

Step One: Recognize the Warning Signs of Heart Disease

The first step in the Heart Smart Program is learning to protect yourself. In Step One you will find out all about chest pain, heart attacks, and the deadly process of atherosclerosis that causes coronary heart disease—and how to recognize the first signs of trouble.

In chapter 1 you'll read about patients who have lived through heart attacks. You'll also hear from them firsthand about the warning signs they had as well as get their advice on how to act and react during a heart attack—and survive it.

Chapter 2, "The Ultimate Chest Pain Guide," will help you sort out the dangerous from the not-so-dangerous causes of chest pain and keep you from panicking every time you feel some pain in your chest.

In chapter 3, we'll look at the underlying cause of heart attacks and coronary heart disease: atherosclerosis, the complex process that is your number-one enemy.

Step Two: Take Charge of Your Cardiac Risk Factors

Once you understand what to watch out for, it's time to start digging into your personal cardiac risk. Step Two of the Heart Smart Program tells you how to take charge of your cardiac risk factors.

Chapters 4 through 6 take an in-depth, comprehensive look at how to test for, identify, *and treat* the traditional cardiac risk factors that cause most heart attacks, strokes, and coronary heart disease. Those are high blood pressure, the "new" diabetes, smoking, obesity, a sedentary lifestyle, high LDL (bad) cholesterol, low HDL (good) cholesterol, and high triglycerides.

Step Three: Go High-Tech to Detect Heart Disease and Lower Your Risk

At long last, emerging cardiovascular technology is focused on detecting heart disease in its *earliest* stages. Believe it or not, new tests can detect heart disease *before* symptoms develop, not after. In Step Three of the Heart Smart Program, I cover all the new, "emerging" cardiac risk factors, the new lab tests, and the multimillion-dollar high-tech imaging studies that currently provide new resources for heart disease prevention and detection. This very exciting step tells you about the latest and greatest tools available to help you determine your cardiac risk and prevent heart attacks.

In chapter 7 you will learn how to avoid being the next "completely healthy" victim of a stealthy heart attack. From C-reactive protein levels to assessing the size and amount of your bad cholesterol, find out which emerging cardiac risk factors you may need to be tested for.

Chapter 8 is the *only source* for finding out the truth about stress testing. Stress tests are a valuable tool in our fight against coronary heart disease, but this chapter makes you aware of the potential downsides of stress testing that can leave you at high risk for a heart attack.

Chapter 9 offers a firsthand look at the new era of high-tech preventive cardiology. You'll read how breakthroughs in imaging quality and technique now provide us with unprecedented opportunities to look inside our arteries noninvasively to detect heart disease at its earliest stages and to predict with accuracy our risk of a heart attack.

By reading this section of the book you'll learn definitively whether you should have one of these tests as part of your program to prevent heart disease.

Step Four: Putting It All Together: What's Your Risk?

Step Four gives you everything you need to know to easily calculate your personal risk. You'll learn how to use your traditional risk factors, emerging risk factors, and the high-tech tests from Steps Two and Three to estimate your risk for coronary heart disease.

Step Five: Live the Heart Smart Life: A Cardiologist's Practical and Proven Approach

Step Five of the Heart Smart Program introduces you to a no-nonsense, straightforward, proven, and effective strategy to prevent, treat, and reverse coronary heart disease. Being Heart Smart encompasses all aspects of your life. It's about making exercise and fitness a major priority. It's about choosing foods that are good for your heart and don't cause obesity.

Kick off your new heart-healthy lifestyle in chapter 11 by learning the 101 action items you can do right now to stop or prevent coronary heart disease. Then dive into what may be one of the most important elements in my program: exercise. In chapter 12 you'll discover how exercise can single-handedly lower your risk of cardiovascular disease and diabetes as well as lower your blood pressure, lower your cholesterol, help you lose weight, improve your bone strength, make you happier, and improve the way you look.

Next we'll turn to the central role nutrition and diet play in living a Heart Smart life. In chapter 13 you will read about the good fats, the bad fats, and a cardiologist's take on the Atkins, the South Beach, and the Mediterranean diets. In addition, you will be introduced to the cardiac "superfoods" such as nuts, fish, soy, and fiber. Finally, in chapter 14 find out which life-saving medications you may not be able to live without.

Don't Be a Victim: Take Charge of Your Heart Health

If you wait for your doctor, or for your spouse or your children, to take control of your heart health and cardiac risk factors, it will be *too late*. Unfortunately, millions of people have cholesterol building up in their heart arteries right now but they simply don't know it, and those completely silent blockages put them at high risk for heart attacks.

With this book you will understand the weaknesses of our current approach to heart disease prevention and treatment and discover the new technology and medicines that are ready to catapult us into a new era of early detection and prevention. Armed with this knowledge, you can take charge of your health and protect yourself from disabling heart attacks or premature cardiac death.

It is never too late to become heart smart!

STEP ONE

Recognize the Warning Signs of Heart Disease

A heart attack feels *nothing* like you thought one would. All the heart attack victims I've ever known have told me that their symptoms were not at all what they had imagined.

But if the symptoms you experience don't feel the way you expected them to, how will you know when to be worried or when to get help? Making the right decisions when you're having chest pain is serious business—life-and-death business. You have to act quickly, and you have to take the right steps: there's no time to do an Internet search for information, and there's no time to phone a friend for advice. Chest pain requires prompt, life-saving action, with no excuses and no delays.

If chest pain hits, will you know what to do? Are you willing to *bet your life* that you'll be able to tell the difference between chest pain that comes from your stomach, esophagus, or chest wall muscles, and the life-threatening chest pain that comes from a heart attack?

Step One of the Heart Smart Program is going to give you all the tools you need to recognize the warning signs and symptoms of a heart attack. More importantly, you'll learn how to act and react in order to survive.

Chapter 1

Heart Attack!

Know the Warning Signs to Save Your Life

Robert was only fifty-two years old when he died. His wife was still in shock shortly after his death when she told me what had happened.

I knew something was wrong when Robert came inside after cutting the grass. He was pale, sweating like crazy, and had left the lawn mower running outside. He just plopped down on the couch and asked me to get him a glass of water.

Those were his last words to me. By the time I came back just a few minutes later he was dead.

Robert's tragic story is by no means unique. Three hundred thousand Americans die within the first hour of the onset of a heart attack each year.

But many deaths could be prevented if the victims knew what to do and immediately took action. If Robert was anything like most of my patients in their fifties, he probably kept mowing the lawn for another five, ten, or even fifteen minutes *after* his chest pain started. If he had recognized the *early warning signs* of a heart attack and called 911 immediately, there is a good chance the paramedics would have gotten to his house in time to save his life.

What Exactly Is a Heart Attack?

A heart attack, or myocardial infarction, occurs when the supply of blood and oxygen to a part of your heart muscle becomes blocked. The blockage is caused by a combination of clot and cholesterol inside your heart artery. Since your heart muscle requires a constant supply of fresh blood and oxygen to keep pumping blood to every part of your body, a heart attack is a life-threatening event.

When blood and oxygen are abruptly cut off during a heart attack, the heart reacts badly. In fact, if it goes without blood and oxygen for more than about ten or fifteen minutes, the heart muscle begins to die. If the blocked heart artery is not treated and opened quickly, the affected part of the heart muscle dies and is permanently replaced by scar tissue, preventing it from functioning fully.

Heart attacks can lead to dangerous arrhythmias and congestive heart failure, and can even result in sudden cardiac death.

Small vs. Large Heart Attack

When it comes to heart attacks, size matters. The size and extent of your heart attack help determine your prognosis.

Two major factors decide whether you had a large heart attack or a small one: the location of the blockage and the duration of the blockage.

Location, Location, Location

The location of the clot plays a big role in determining the size and severity of a heart attack. Clots that occur in larger vessels and clots that occur farther upstream in your heart artery lead to a larger heart attack and more damage. If the blockage takes place in a smaller branch vessel, only a small part of the heart muscle will be affected.

Blockage Duration

The second factor that determines the size and severity of your heart attack is how long the artery is blocked. The longer the artery remains choked off, the more heart damage is done. This is the reason you must act so quickly at the first sign of trouble.

Each additional minute your heart artery remains blocked increases your chances of sustaining life-threatening heart arrhythmias and becoming chronically disabled. The heart is not at all forgiving.

The best way to minimize heart attack damage is to call 911 as soon as you have chest pain.

How Big Was Your Heart Attack?

If you've had a heart attack and don't know if it was a large or a small one, ask your doctor about your Ejection Fraction, or EF. The Ejection Fraction tells you the percentage of blood your heart pump ejects with each beat; in other words it is a measure of how strong your heart pump is. A normal EF is 55 to 70 percent. Your EF is one of the best ways to predict how well you will recover after a heart attack and learn how much damage the heart attack did to your heart. (Your doctor can determine your EF through a heart angiogram, a heart ultrasound, or a stress test.)

What Are the Warning Signs?

One of my patients summed it up best when he said: *"It was really strange, I never felt any of the severe pain I expected during my heart attack. There was clearly an uncomfortable crushing feeling across my chest and I felt a little sweaty, but that's about it. There was no pain at all."*

Almost one in four heart attack victims misinterprets his or her heart attack symptoms as being caused by something else. This is a costly, often fatal mistake that you can avoid by knowing what to look for.

While many heart attack symptoms vary from person to person, there are some that most people share. Not every person will suffer these classic symptoms, but the vast majority of heart attack victims feel at least one of them.

Chest Pain (or Chest "Discomfort")

The most common symptom caused by a heart attack is chest pain. But different patients feel the pain differently. Chest pain has been experienced by heart attack victims as

- Heaviness, tightness, squeezing, or pressure
- Pain that is located in the left side of the chest but that may radiate to the left *or* right shoulder and arm, neck, jaw, teeth, ear, or back
- Pain that starts suddenly, while you're at rest or with exertion
- Chest discomfort that is constant and lasts for more than ten to fifteen minutes

- Chest discomfort that is hard to pinpoint: it might be in the middle of the chest or "all over" the chest

In their own words, victims have described heart attacks in these ways:

- "There is an elephant (or weight or brick) sitting on my chest."
- "It feels like a band being tightened around my chest."
- "I can't pinpoint the symptoms but it's just uncomfortable inside my chest rather than a pain."
- "There is a tightness in my chest and around my heart."
- "It feels like a heavy pressure on the chest."
- "It feels like someone has a hand on my heart and is squeezing it."

Beyond Chest Pain

Chest pain or pressure may be your only warning sign of a heart attack, but it's more likely you'll feel a constellation of symptoms:

- Shortness of breath
- Difficulty breathing
- Feeling cold and clammy
- Sweating
- Extreme weakness, fatigue, or exhaustion
- Nausea or vomiting
- Palpitations or fluttering in the chest
- Dizziness or light-headedness

Heart Smart Chest Pain Alert!

Women, diabetics, and senior citizens often do not experience *any* of the classic heart attack symptoms. Fatigue, palpitations, and vague chest pain may be the only warning signs.

The "Classic" Heart Attack

The following is a typical heart attack scenario. If you find yourself having a similar experience, call for help immediately.

You are sitting at the dinner table when all of a sudden you feel a pressure or heaviness in either the middle or the left side of your chest. It may be very diffi-cult to pinpoint the exact location of the discomfort, but it feels heavy and uncom-fortable "inside" your chest.

The pressure or heaviness quickly grows stronger as your heart muscle cells begin to die. The chest discomfort may start to spread to your jaw, neck, teeth, ear, or either arm. The pain in those areas has a similar "heaviness" to the chest dis-comfort you feel.

You begin to feel weak and break out in a cold sweat. A touch of nausea creeps in. Now you start to think that something is dreadfully wrong. You even begin to think that maybe you really are having a heart attack. But then you tell yourself "It can't be" because you have never had any symptoms before. Still, the feeling is different from the acid reflux symptoms you've had and any other discomfort or pain you have experienced. You go back and forth in your mind as to what could be causing this heaviness and pressure in your chest.

While you are trying to figure out what is going on, your wife (or husband) tells you that you look pale and clammy. Your spouse wants to know what is wrong. At this point you must make a decision. Either you lie and say, "Noth-ing," that you just need to rest for a while, or you do the right thing and say you are having a heart attack and that 911 should be called.

Calling 911 can save your life.

Heart Attack Survival Guide

The scenario above, and others very much like it, take place more than a million times a year across the United States. Familiarizing yourself with the symptoms and the progression of a heart attack will enable you to act correctly and immediately if you experience one.

But what *is* the right thing to do?

How you *react to heart attack symptoms* is just as important as recog-nizing them. If you have *any* of the above symptoms or even consider that you might be having a heart attack, you need to act immediately. Fear, hesitation, and doubt lead to *fatal delays* in treatment.

Six Steps to Take Instantly

1. Stop what you are doing and lie down.

2. Don't panic.

3. Direct someone to call 911 and to say that you are having a heart attack.

4. If they're available, chew a full-strength aspirin or two "baby" aspirin.

5. If one is available, place a nitroglycerine tablet under your tongue.

6. If you can, ask someone near you if an automatic external defibrillator (AED) is available (these are now found in many public places). If not, ask if anyone nearby knows CPR—just in case.

Six Mistakes to Avoid

1. Downplay or ignore your symptoms.

2. Delay seeking help because of fear or embarrassment that your symptoms might not mean you're having a heart attack.

3. Try driving yourself to the emergency room.

4. Think you're too young or too healthy to have a heart attack.

5. Think that since you are a woman you could not be having a heart attack, that only men have heart attacks.

6. Delay medical care because you do not want to bother your spouse/parent/children/neighbors.

Don't Make Up Excuses

Evelyn lived alone on a quiet cul-de-sac surrounded by mostly elderly neighbors and friends. One night after dinner, she had a sudden onset of chest heaviness and pressure in her mid and upper chest.

Evelyn's initial instincts were right on target. She recognized that her symptoms were likely due to a heart attack and she thought she should call 911. But that's when her chest pain excuse kicked in. If she called 911 she feared her elderly neighbors would become very upset when they saw an ambulance come to her house, and she didn't want to upset them.

Evelyn never did call 911. Instead, after much consternation and many precious minutes, she called her daughter, who came right over and immediately called 911. But the twenty-five-minute delay was too long.

Evelyn died needlessly that night because her fear of upsetting her neighbors overrode her recognition of her symptoms and her correct instinct to call for help.

Making excuses or downplaying your symptoms is not a Heart Smart decision. I've heard all sorts of crazy reasons why patients didn't call for help as soon as they started having a heart attack—from not wanting to miss a business luncheon to not wanting to leave their dog home alone. These excuses all cost these patients precious time. Here are some excuses that should *not* keep you from calling 911 if you think you're having a heart attack:

- It's probably just indigestion.
- I don't want to spend the next three hours in the emergency room.
- I don't want to call 911 if it's not really a heart attack.
- I will be embarrassed if it turns out to be something other than my heart.
- I don't want anyone to worry about me.
- It can't be a heart attack because I've never had any other symptoms.

Heart Attack Survivor Secrets

Heart attack survivors get it right. They make the right decisions at the right times. There are *major action differences* between people who survive a heart attack and people who don't. Here are a few heart attack survivor secrets:

- Heart attack survivors recognize the *early* warning signs and symptoms of a heart attack.
- Heart attack survivors call 911 without delay.
- Heart attack survivors get help first and worry about the consequences later.
- Heart attack survivors don't make excuses or downplay symptoms.
- Heart attack survivors always err on the side of caution.
- Heart attack survivors would rather spend three hours in the emergency room and find out that their heart is fine than wish they had gone to the emergency room as they slip into unconsciousness.

Summing It Up

A heart attack is a life-threatening medical emergency that must be recognized as soon as symptoms develop. Delays in treating heart attacks lead to congestive heart failure, dangerous cardiac arrhythmias, and sudden cardiac death.

Become a chest pain expert. Being able to recognize the early warning signs and symptoms of a heart attack is your best bet for survival.

Chapter 2

The Ultimate Chest Pain Guide

When Should You Worry?

Have you ever had chest pain? Almost everyone gets some sort of chest pain from time to time. The trick is knowing which is the "don't worry about it" kind of chest pain and which is the "I'm in trouble" kind. The Heart Smart Ultimate Chest Pain Guide will tell you everything you need to know to make the right decision when you have chest pain and to help keep you safe while limiting your stress and anxiety.

Sorting Out the Possibilities

Sorting out chest pain is my life. At the office, in the emergency room, at parties, on the golf course, and even at my dry cleaner's, everyone tells me about their chest pain. It's practically a given that soon after a new acquaintance finds out I'm a cardiologist, I'll hear, "You know, I get this chest pain when . . ."

That's okay with me. Chest pain can be a very scary thing, especially when you don't know why you're having it. And it can be difficult to know why you're having it, since chest pain can come not only from your heart but also from your stomach, a strained muscle, even stress and strong emotions such as anger, anxiety, and extreme sadness.

Chest Pain Diagnosis Challenges

Pinpointing where chest pain is coming from can be challenging, for doctors as well as for patients. That's because:

- There's a lot going on in the chest area. Muscles, tendons, joints, the lungs, the heart, esophagus, stomach, and aorta all make their home in the chest cavity—and they can all cause chest pain.

- Many of the structures in the chest cavity share nerve pathways. That means all of them cause a similar type of pain when things go wrong. It's also the reason you experience referred pain—pain that moves from one area to another (as in heart attack pain that goes to the arm).

- Everyone has his or her unique perception of pain as well as a unique level of pain tolerance. The same condition could cause you to feel pressure but cause someone else to feel something like a sharp poke.

- Some causes of chest pain are serious life-threatening problems, while others are completely benign. So you always have to err on the side of caution.

Details Help Make the Determination

When you have chest pain, your doctor will need to know a lot of details to figure out what's causing it. Common questions you'll likely be asked include:

- What does the pain feel like?
- When does the pain come on?
- How long does the pain last—seconds, minutes, hours, or days?
- Does it get worse when you eat or exercise?
- Does a certain position relieve the pain or make it worse?
- Does taking nitroglycerin lessen the pain?

The doctor will also want to know your age and your overall cardiac risk (see Step Four for help determining your risk). Being able to provide your doctor with these details will dramatically improve his or her chances of quickly diagnosing and treating your chest pain.

Causes of Chest Pain

I like to break the different causes of chest pain down into two categories: life-threatening and everything else.

Life-Threatening Causes of Chest Pain

Heart attacks, angina, aortic dissection, and pulmonary embolism are the four most common life-threatening causes of chest pain. Here is a description of each as well as their common symptoms.

Heart attack: A sudden onset of heaviness, pressure, squeezing, or tightness across the chest.

Chest pain that results from a heart attack must be recognized and acted upon immediately.

Angina: Crushing chest pressure and shortness of breath with exertion, relieved with rest.

Angina is chest pain or pressure caused by blockages in the heart artery that limit the amount of blood that gets to your heart muscle. During times of activity your heart muscle pumps harder and faster, requiring more fuel in the form of oxygen delivered in the blood by the heart artery. If the artery is blocked, the heart muscle won't receive the blood and oxygen it needs to meet the increased demand. So the starving heart muscle cells scream out for more blood, causing chest pain known as angina.

Because of your heart's amazing built-in "reserves," by the time your heart artery is no longer able to keep up with your heart muscle's demands for more oxygen, your heart artery is already more than 70 percent blocked. That means that by the time you have angina, you already have severe, advanced coronary artery disease.

A heart attack and angina are closely related, but there is an important difference between the two. During a heart attack, the heart artery completely closes; the pain comes from the heart muscle actually dying from lack of oxygen. With angina, the pain comes from the oxygen-deprived heart muscle calling out for help. The muscle is not dead, but it's at risk of dying.

Aortic dissection: A severe tearing or ripping type of chest pain that runs down the chest and back.

Aortic dissection is an uncommon but often fatal cause of chest pain. Actor John Ritter's tragic and early death from aortic dissection put this killer condition into the spotlight. Early recognition of its symptoms is critical for improving your chances of survival.

An aortic dissection is a tear in the wall of the aorta, the largest artery in the body. You may be at high risk for aortic dissection if you have hypertension and/or if you smoke cigarettes. People with connective-tissue diseases such as Marfan's syndrome are also at increased risk for aortic dissection.

The pain typically associated with aortic dissection is unique: it is a sudden onset of severe chest pain that often radiates to the back and shoulders. The chest pain is usually sharp, and victims often use words such as "tearing" or "ripping" to describe it. That description is right on target. An aortic dissection can tear the aorta from the base of the heart all the way down to the arteries of the legs.

Some form of chest and back pain is present in almost all cases of aortic dissection. But additional symptoms are common as well, including nausea, passing out, shortness of breath, and leg pain. Symptoms will vary depending on where the tear starts and where it ends.

Aortic dissection is a life-threatening emergency. If you feel a sharp, tearing pain in your chest and back, call 911 immediately.

Pulmonary embolism: A sharp type of chest pain that gets worse when you take a deep breath; accompanied by shortness of breath.

A pulmonary embolism (PE) is a very common and highly lethal condition that is a leading cause of death in the United States. It is not really a disease, but an often-fatal complication of an underlying disease called *venous thrombosis*. You may be at high risk for a PE if you recently had surgery or recently were or are now pregnant, are immobilized for a prolonged period, or have an underlying cancer.

When your body is healthy, small clots form throughout your veins to help protect you from bleeding. But the above conditions cause this clotting process to get out of hand and result in the formation of large clots. A pulmonary embolism occurs when one of these clots breaks off from within a vein in your arm or leg and travels to the pulmonary arteries in your lungs. There it lodges and obstructs the blood flow, basically causing a "lung attack" as opposed to a heart attack.

When this lung attack occurs, you experience the symptoms of the PE. The three most classic symptoms are chest pain, shortness of breath, and hemoptysis. The chest pain from a PE is described as a sharp, stabbing pain and often gets much worse when you take a deep breath. The pain may also radiate to your shoulder or back. If hemoptysis occurs it means you are coughing up blood-tinged sputum.

A variety of less common symptoms can also be associated with PEs. These include passing out, abdominal pain, fever, cough, and a racing heart.

Recognizing the risks as well as the symptoms of PE can help save your life. Of the half a million deaths from PE each year in the United States, more than a hundred thousand of the victims could have survived with prompt diagnosis and treatment.

Less Dangerous Causes of Chest Pain

Most chest pain is more of a nuisance than a life-threatening medical problem. Learning to recognize the symptoms of these common causes of chest pain will help lower your anxiety level when the pain occurs.

The two most common sources of chest pain are the musculoskeletal and gastrointestinal systems. Anxiety, stress, or irritation of the sac around your heart also can lead to chest pain and discomfort.

Musculoskeletal-caused chest pain: Sharp or nagging chest pain—there are no other symptoms—that can be pinpointed with your finger; certain positions may relieve or worsen the pain.

Musculoskeletal pain is the term used for pain that comes from the muscles, tendons, joints, and bones in the chest wall, shoulders, neck, and back. Musculoskeletal problems are the most common causes of chest pain.

Chest pain from a musculoskeletal injury may show up immediately with an injury or even occur a day or two after you injured yourself. Twisting, turning, bending, stretching, lifting, pushing, and pulling can all take their toll on the musculoskeletal system. Irritation and inflammation of the musculoskeletal system also can be caused by overexertion, taking part in activities that involve repetitive motions, and from overdoing exercise on weekends.

Chest pain from a musculoskeletal injury usually is described as sharp, stabbing, or knifelike. The most classic feature of a musculoskeletal injury is pain that becomes worse when you activate the inflamed or affected area.

Musculoskeletal chest pain often can be triggered by touching a "sore spot" and can be pinpointed with one finger. Getting into a certain position, for example, and raising your arm also may bring on the chest pain. The pain may bother you only while doing certain activities, or it may last for hours or even days at a time

To treat musculoskeletal chest pain, rest and avoid movements that involve the affected area of the body. Anti-inflammatory medications also may be used to relieve persistent pain.

Gastrointestinal-caused chest pain: Chest pain caused by irritation of the esophagus, stomach, or gallbladder.

Gastroesophageal reflux disease (GERD):   Burning discomfort from the middle of the chest up to the throat, which may be worse when you lie in bed at night or after eating certain foods.

Gastroesophageal reflux, also known as acid reflux or heartburn, is a common condition that affects eighteen million people chronically in the United States. GERD is caused by stomach acid that leaks out of the stomach and backs up into the esophagus. While the stomach has a protective lining that prevents the acid from damaging it, the esophagus does not have a protective coat. Over time, GERD can cause significant damage to the lining of the esophagus and even cancer.

GERD commonly causes chest pain and discomfort. The pain usually is described as burning or a heatlike sensation, but some people feel it more as pressure or heaviness in the chest. The discomfort occurs in the mid to upper chest behind the breastbone. Belching, "gas" pains, and an acid taste in the back of the throat are other symptoms associated with GERD.

GERD symptoms are more commonly experienced at night when you're lying flat in bed or after eating a spicy or greasy meal. Late-night meals, caffeine, tea, cola, chocolate, tobacco, spicy foods, onions, and alcohol all can exacerbate your symptoms. Unlike chest pain from a heart attack or angina, chest pain from GERD is usually not related to exertion.

Medications and, rarely, surgical intervention can sometimes improve GERD symptoms. But making lifestyle changes, including losing weight, eating smaller meals, getting regular exercise, and avoiding the above triggers can significantly improve symptoms. If lifestyle changes don't resolve your symptoms, your doctor may prescribe antacids, H-2 blockers, or proton pump inhibitors. Because GERD can cause dangerous complications over time, always let your doctor know if you experience any symptoms.

Gallbladder disease: Sharp chest pain that starts in the right upper abdomen and may travel to your right shoulder; chest pain becomes worse after greasy meals and can last for hours.

Gallstones are another common cause of chest pain. You are at risk for gallstones if you are overweight, in your forties, female, or have high cholesterol.

The gallbladder stores bile made in the liver that is used to help digest fat. When gallstones form they block the bile from being released, causing a buildup of pressure inside the gallbladder. This increased pressure causes a colicky type of chest pain and abdominal pain that develops over an hour and lasts for a few hours. The pain may radiate up to the right shoulder blade or between the shoulder blades.

An acute gallbladder attack that involves a fever and severe pain is a surgical emergency. Nonsurgical treatment includes avoiding eating greasy, fatty foods.

Esophageal spasm: Tightness or squeezing in the midchest that is not related to exertion or activity.

The esophagus is a muscle-lined tube that transports food from your mouth to your stomach. Esophageal spasms occur when the muscles lining the esophagus go into spasm.

The pain caused by esophageal spasm is very similar to pain caused by a heart attack: there's a heaviness or tightness in the mid to upper chest right behind the breastbone. The discomfort also may radiate to the arm or the jaw.

It is virtually impossible for you to tell the difference between the pain from a heart attack and the pain from esophageal spasm—esophageal spasm is the great heart attack imitator. So don't try to sort it out. Get to the emergency room and let the doctors figure it out for you.

There are no clear triggers or risk factors for esophageal spasm. Some tests are available to diagnose it, but they are not very accurate, so doctors tend not to use them but to treat the condition. Treatment involves using some of the same medications that treat heart disease. Nitroglycerin and calcium channel blockers help relax the smooth muscle around your esophagus to relieve symptoms.

Other Common Causes of Chest Pain

Anxiety and stress: The strong responses to difficult or emotional situations.

Anxiety, stress, and emotional distress—which affect everyone from time to time—can cause chest pain or a feeling of tightness around the heart. While the symptoms occur during stressful times, they have no relation to activity level or exercise. In fact, many people think exercise *helps* this type of chest pain.

Headache, stomach irritability, palpitations, hyperventilation, and even full-blown panic attacks can accompany stress-induced chest pain.

Chest pain caused by stress or anxiety can feel very much like pain caused by a heart attack. So always err on the side of caution and assume the worst if you are not sure where your pain is coming from.

Pericarditis: Sharp, jabbing pain around the heart made worse by lying flat and improved by sitting up and leaning forward.

Pericarditis is caused by an irritation and inflammation of the sac, or pericardium, that encases your heart. The most common cause of this condition is a viral infection, although many times no exact cause is found.

The chest pain associated with pericarditis is sharp or stabbing rather than squeezing or a feeling of pressure. It occurs in the midchest area around the heart. The pain often radiates up to the left shoulder and to the back. Other symptoms, such as shortness of breath, fever, and sweats, often accompany the chest pain.

The most classic feature of pericarditis pain is that it is worse when you lie flat on your back and is relieved when you sit or lean forward. Leaning forward draws the inflamed pericardial sac away from surrounding structures, limiting the inflammation.

Pericarditis is treated with anti-inflammatory medications such as indomethacin and steroids. Symptoms usually resolve quickly, and the outcome and prognosis generally are excellent.

Figuring Out the Cause

Correctly diagnosing chest pain is critical to your survival—and too important for you to take on by yourself. The following guide will help you recognize your symptoms. But always let your doctor know when you have chest pain so he or she can diagnose and treat it.

Chest Pain Guide

	Heart Attack and Angina	GI-Related*	Musculoskeletal	Pericarditis
Description of Chest Pain	Tightness, pressure, squeezing, or heaviness	Burning, acidlike, hot	Achy, sharp, dull, knifelike	Sharp, jabbing
Location	Midchest, hard to pinpoint	Middle of chest, up and down	Anywhere across chest	Midchest

	Heart Attack and Angina	GI-Related*	Musculoskeletal	Pericarditis
Radiates to	Left or right arm, neck, jaw, back	Stomach, abdomen	Shoulder, back, neck, arms	Back, shoulder
Duration	Longer than 10–15 minutes, may come in waves	Hours	Constant for days or related to particular position	Constant for days
Things That Make the Pain Worse	Any exertion	Lying flat, eating a meal (pain worsens after meal)	Motion of upper body, pressing on it	Lying back, coughing, breathing deeply
Things That Make the Pain Better	Nitroglycerin, rest	Antacids	Rubbing it, changing position, anti-inflammatory medication	Sitting up and leaning forward, anti-inflammatory medication

*GI = Gastrointestinal

Chest Pain Diagnostic Tests

If the cause of your chest pain is not obvious, your physician may order tests to help make a diagnosis. Tests range from the quick and easy EKG to the invasive heart angiogram.

Electrocardiogram (EKG)   An EKG is a simple test that is routinely used as the first step in evaluating chest pain. Angina, heart attack, and heart arrhythmia can all be detected quickly and accurately with an EKG. During an EKG, sensors are placed on your chest to "listen" to and record the electrical activity of your heart. The test is painless and takes about five minutes to perform.

Cardiac stress test   Stress tests are a critical component of the chest pain evaluation. Stress tests, through exercise or medications, allow your doctor to put your heart under stress by increasing its need for oxygen. During a stress test an EKG and oftentimes some type of imaging procedure, such as an echocardiogram, monitor your heart.

A stress test immediately sorts out whether your symptoms are heart-related. If the results of your stress test are normal, that indicates that your chest pain is not heart-related. If you fail the test, your pain is due to coronary artery disease (see chapter 8 for all the stress test details).

Heart angiogram   The heart angiogram is another tool for evaluating heart artery blockages. A heart angiogram is an invasive test done in the hospital requiring a catheter tube to be passed through a large artery in your leg up to your heart. Its invasive nature and potential complications make it a last resort for evaluating chest pain unless your doctor is quite suspicious that your chest pain is due to heart artery blockage.

Chest X-ray   A chest X-ray is a great tool for evaluating the lungs and the bony structures of the chest wall. Lung infections, fluid-filled lungs, a "collapsed" lung, and lung cancer are less common causes of chest pain that can readily be detected by a chest X-ray.

Endoscopy   If your chest pain has a decidedly gastrointestinal component, further evaluation with an endoscope may be your first test. Stomach doctors use an endoscope, a special camera attached to a "scope," to look into the esophagus and stomach for problems.

The Triple Rule-out

Coming soon to an emergency room near you is technology that can diagnose three of the most life-threatening causes of chest pain in just a few seconds. The cardiac CT with coronary angiography can rule out aortic dissection, pulmonary embolism, and coronary artery disease in the blink of an eye. This life-saving technology is revolutionizing the way we evaluate and treat people with chest pain (see chapter 9).

Summing It Up

Having chest pain is frightening. Are you having a heart attack, or are you feeling symptoms of one of the less dangerous causes of chest pain?

I don't expect you to be able to figure out the cause of chest pain you experience, but I hope I've been able to clarify the difference between life-threatening causes of chest pain and less worrisome culprits. Read through the symptoms again and keep the Chest Pain Guide handy. They could make the difference between life and death.

The most important thing to remember, however, is that whenever chest pain strikes, don't hesitate to call for help if you think you need it.

Chapter 3

Attack of the Killer Plaque

Coronary Heart Disease and Atherosclerosis

The devastating effects of cardiovascular disease are so common and prevalent that we have become numb to the fact that coronary heart disease is nearly completely preventable.

Fifty years ago, "hardening of the arteries" (actually hard deposits of calcium in cholesterol plaques) and dying from heart disease were considered to be inevitable parts of the aging process, but thanks to the Framingham studies carried out in the early 1960s, we became wise to the fact that risk factors such as smoking and high blood pressure promoted coronary heart disease.

Today we also know that obesity, a sedentary lifestyle, high cholesterol, high blood pressure, and diabetes cause the vast majority of cases of coronary heart disease and almost every heart attack.

In this chapter we're going to look at the underlying process responsible for coronary heart disease, heart attacks, and angina.

What Is Heart Disease?

"Heart disease" is a generic term referring to any disorder that primarily affects your heart. Disorders of the heart valves, abnormal cardiac rhythms, and congenital heart problems can all be lumped into the category of "heart disease."

Most of the time, however, when we say "heart disease" we are actually referring to *coronary* heart disease. Coronary heart disease refers to disease of the arteries of the heart. The arteries that supply the heart with blood and oxygen are the coronary arteries. Coronary heart disease is also known as atherosclerotic heart disease, arteriosclerotic heart disease, and coronary artery disease. No matter what you call it, this condition is a relentless killer.

U.S. Cardiovascular Disease Fact Sheet

In the United States alone, more than 60 million people have some form of cardiovascular disease. The disease

- Is a leading killer of both men and women
- Kills about one million people a year
- Accounts for about half of all deaths each year
- Causes more than 150,000 premature deaths each year
- Kills one out of every three of its victims, with no warning
- Kills 2,600 people each day (1 every 33 seconds)
- Kills more people than the next six causes of death combined (including all types of cancer, accidents, and HIV/AIDS)
- Affects one in ten women 45 to 64 years of age

To keep from becoming another coronary heart disease statistic, it's necessary to know your enemy, how your enemy acts, where your enemy is likely to attack, and your enemy's weaknesses. In the case of coronary heart disease, your primary enemy is atherosclerosis.

Atherosclerosis: Getting to the Core of the Problem

Atherosclerosis is a perhaps unfamiliar word that you will see often in this book. Atherosclerosis is an abnormal *inflammatory process* inside artery walls as the result of complex interactions among "bad" cholesterol (see chapter 6), platelets, calcium, and inflammatory cells.

In *subclinical* atherosclerosis, cholesterol is building up in your arteries but has not declared itself yet in the form of chest pain, a heart attack, or a stroke. If you have had an angioplasty or bypass surgery or suffered a heart attack or a stroke, then you have the *clinical* form of atherosclerosis.

All efforts to prevent as well as treat coronary heart disease are really aimed at preventing, reversing, and halting the atherosclerosis process. That's because if the process goes unchecked and untreated, you will wind up with blocked arteries somewhere in your body; atherosclerosis can take place in arteries anywhere in your body. If a blockage develops in your carotid arteries (the arteries in your neck), you'll have a stroke. If it develops in your coronary arteries, you'll have a heart attack. If one develops in your leg arteries, you'll have leg pain or "claudications."

What Causes Atherosclerosis?

Because atherosclerosis is such a complex inflammatory process, the medical profession doesn't yet completely understand all the mechanics of how it causes blockages. But we do know about most of the things that cause it.

There are two categories of risk factors for atherosclerosis and coronary heart disease: traditional and emerging.

The *traditional risk factors for atherosclerosis* are obesity, smoking, a sedentary lifestyle, high cholesterol, high blood pressure, diabetes, poor dietary habits, a family history of coronary artery disease, and increasing age. Nine out of ten people with atherosclerosis and coronary artery disease have at least one of these traditional cardiac risk factors (see Step Two).

The *emerging risk factors for atherosclerosis* relate more to the inflammatory, infectious, and clotting aspects of the atherosclerotic process rather than to the hereditary and lifestyle aspects. Emerging cardiac risk factors (see chapter 7 for details on this) include high homocysteine levels, some types of infections, elevated clotting factors, and specialized subcomponents of cholesterol.

With a little bit of detective work along with use of state-of-the-art imaging and testing techniques, your doctor can determine your particular risks for atherosclerosis and get you on the road to preventing or treating the disease.

When Does Atherosclerosis Begin?

Believe it or not, atherosclerosis rears its ugly head while you are still in school. Not graduate school, not college, but high school or even middle school. The process starts early and continues its silent attack for decades.

A number of studies have been done specifically to look at when and how atherosclerosis begins. The Pathobiological Determinants of

Atherosclerosis in Youth study, or PDAY, reported in the *Journal of the American Medical Association* that children as young as fifteen years commonly experience the early stages of atherosclerosis. The study showed that kids who were obese or had elevated LDL cholesterol levels (see chapter 6) were more likely to have developed the disease. Another study, the Muscatine study, published in the American Heart Association's scientific journal *Circulation*, reported that obesity, high blood pressure, and low HDL cholesterol levels were associated with coronary atherosclerosis in adolescents and young adults.

Stages of Atherosclerosis

There are five stages of atherosclerosis. Of course, your goal should be to stop and stabilize the atherosclerotic process in the earliest stage possible in order to accomplish your goal of staying heart healthy. Many of you will be able to prevent the first phase of atherosclerosis from taking place, while most of you will be trying to reverse stages 2, 3, or 4. Progressing through the five stages of atherosclerosis is slow and complex and usually takes decades to occur.

The five stages of atherosclerosis are

1. Breakdown of the inner layer of the arteries' defense system
2. Invasion of the artery wall by LDL cholesterol
3. A nasty and complex local inflammatory reaction
4. The formation of cholesterol "plaque"
5. The rupture of the plaque, resulting in a heart attack and sometimes death

Stage 1. Endothelial Dysfunction: Your Shield Is Broken

Your body's first line of defense against the attack of cholesterol is the inner lining of your heart artery wall. If this arterial wall shield holds strong, your heart artery stays almost impervious to attack. If your shield breaks, though, you become at high risk for a successful cholesterol attack.

The walls of your arteries are composed of three distinct layers: the *intima*, the *media*, and the *adventitia*. The inner intima layer is lined by a thin layer of cells called the *endothelium*, which is in contact with the blood circulating in the arteries.

Because it is so tiny and thin, the endothelium is an unlikely primary defense shield. But a healthy, happy endothelium will protect you from attack by dangerous LDL cholesterol that's circulating in your blood. The endothelium guards the gate to the local defense system and to the overall health of the arterial wall.

An unhealthy, or *dysfunctional*, endothelium puts your heart artery at high risk for invasion. Once this shield is punctured, only bad things can happen.

What Breaks the Shield? There's no mystery about what causes endothelial dysfunction. The most common causes of endothelial dysfunction are

- High levels of LDL, or "bad," cholesterol
- Low levels of HDL, or "good," cholesterol
- Cigarette smoking
- Uncontrolled diabetes mellitus
- High blood pressure
- Inherited/genetic factors

No matter which condition causes the arterial wall shield to break, you will not know it has broken because no symptoms are associated with endothelial dysfunction.

How Do I Know if I Have Endothelial Dysfunction?

Even though there are no visible symptoms of the breakdown of the endothelium, you can determine if this has happened to you. A noninvasive test called the brachial artery reactivity test can detect endothelial dysfunction and help predict your risk for cardiovascular disease. See chapter 9 for details.

Stage 2. The LDL Cholesterol Invasion

LDL cholesterol is the villain of the second stage of atherosclerosis. Because the endothelium was pierced in stage 1, you are now susceptible to an all-out attack from bad LDL cholesterol. While high levels of LDL cholesterol are especially dangerous, *even LDL cholesterol at normal levels* can invade your heart artery and promote atherosclerosis.

What happens in stage 2? LDL cholesterol takes full advantage of the dysfunctional endothelium and wiggles its way from your bloodstream into the inner layer of your arterial wall. Once past your initial defense system, LDL cholesterol has free rein to begin a series of chain reactions and complex interactions that may ultimately result in a heart attack.

Once LDL cholesterol invades your heart artery, you officially have coronary artery disease. And just as in stage 1, you still will not have any symptoms during stage 2 of atherosclerosis

Stage 3. Inflammation and Clotting: Misery Loves Company

Now the plot thickens—things turn from bad to worse. LDL cholesterol continues to invade your heart artery, but, in a strange turn of events, your own body joins the attack by turning against you as well.

Because it has been breached, your damaged endothelium can no longer function normally. Instead of protecting your heart, it now promotes further damage inside the artery. After letting in the LDL cholesterol, it decreases its production of nitric oxide, which causes your arteries to constrict rather than relax in response to injury; this is particularly dangerous during the later stages of atherosclerosis, when the artery is partially blocked. The damaged endothelium also promotes the release of dangerous free radicals from LDL cholesterol, which encourages further damage to the artery wall.

With so much happening, you heart artery becomes confused and struggles to fight off the invasion. It responds by activating blood-clotting factors and sending out messengers to attract inflammatory markers to the area, including monocytes and macrophages (these specialized immune cells are sent to the area of invasion to "gobble up" the foreign invaders).

The bottom line is that the body's response to the LDL invasion of the endothelium actually causes more harm than good. Clotting, constriction of the arteries, and a massive inflammatory response at the site where the endothelium was damaged lead to the earliest form of atherosclerosis, called the *fatty streak*.

But still there are no symptoms of the disease.

Heart Smart Tip

We now know that inflammation plays a key role in heart disease and heart attacks. Many of the new blood tests used for the early prediction of coronary heart disease and atherosclerosis, such as the C-reactive protein (CRP) test, can detect your body's response to the inflammation. See Step Three for more on the latest testing technology for early heart disease detection.

Stage 4. Plaque Formation: Your Last Chance to Stop the Disease

If you reach stage 4 of atherosclerosis, you're in a real danger zone. You can still stop the disease and reverse the damage before you have a heart attack, but you have to do it now.

At this point in the atherosclerosis progression, clotting and other factors have come together to form a more organized entity called fibrous plaque. Fibrous plaque, or cholesterol plaque, is made up of a core pocket of cholesterol-rich foam cells covered by a fibrous "cap" made from connective tissue. Once it has taken this form, the plaque can grow and extend from the inner lining of the heart artery into the lumen, or channel of the artery. As it continues to grow there, it begins to obstruct the artery, limiting blood flow and oxygen to the beating heart muscle.

There are two types of cholesterol plaque: stable and unstable.

Stable plaques have a firm cap covering them, so their inner core of cholesterol, inflammatory agents, and clotting factors does not become directly exposed to the blood. Stable plaques grow slowly over time and eventually will cause symptoms of chest pain. Stable plaques are less likely to rupture suddenly and cause a heart attack. They are often infiltrated with hard deposits of calcium, hence the term "hardening of the arteries."

Unstable plaques are seriously dangerous. These types of plaque are precursors to chest pain, heart attacks, and sudden death. Unstable plaques have only thin, flimsy caps covering their tops, which puts them at high risk of rupturing. If an unstable plaque ruptures, its cholesterol (or lipid) core will reach the blood, causing a severe and overwhelming clotting reaction that leads to a heart attack.

The difference between having a stable and an unstable plaque in your arteries is literally the difference between life and death

In stage 4 you may finally develop some symptoms, the most common of which are chest pain and/or shortness of breath—but you still may not notice any symptoms.

Heart Smart Tip

Some of the new technology reviewed in the Heart Smart Program (see chapter 9) is directed at not only detecting the early formation of plaque but also at differentiating between a stable and an unstable plaque.

Stage 5. Plaque Rupture: Heart Attack and Sometimes Death

You never want to make it to the final phase of atherosclerosis. Stage 5 is better known as a heart attack.

Because unstable plaques are exactly that—unstable—sooner or later something has to give. In the last stage of atherosclerosis, the protective fibrous cap that overlays the plaque's gooey core of cholesterol breaks, causing all the contents of the plaque to spill out into the heart artery. When those contents get mixed into the bloodstream, a massive reaction occurs—extensive clotting and inflammation. The contents of the ruptured plaque completely block the heart artery, resulting in a heart attack.

Now—too late—you finally have symptoms of atherosclerosis.

A Paradigm Shift in Detecting Coronary Heart Disease

For decades, all the progress made in cardiovascular medicine was in treating severe, advanced coronary artery disease. New catheters, balloons, and stents made it possible to open blocked arteries even in the middle of a heart attack. New surgical equipment and techniques made it possible to routinely bypass severely blocked heart arteries.

But all of these advances focused on treating *clinical* atherosclerosis—atherosclerosis that has developed to the point where victims experience one or more symptoms.

Now we're experiencing a shift in the focus of cardiovascular medicine research and development. The spotlight is on finding ways to discover coronary artery disease in its earliest stages—*before* symptoms occur.

Learning that they have *subclinical* atherosclerosis will allow patients to ramp up their efforts to prevent the devastating effects of heart disease. Just as important, learning that they don't have atherosclerosis may prevent them from taking unnecessary medication.

The paradigm shift from working to detect clinical atherosclerosis to working to uncover subclinical atherosclerosis is revolutionizing our ability to effectively prevent coronary heart disease.

It's Not Only a Man's Problem: Women and Coronary Heart Disease

Until the past few years, women were largely ignored when it came to understanding and preventing coronary heart disease. Women were rarely part of clinical trials, they were treated less aggressively than men, and they were tested less often than men.

All that is changing. The American Heart Association is now leading a "Go Red for Women" campaign to raise awareness about coronary artery disease in women. In fact, coronary heart disease is the leading killer of women in the United States; one in ten American women age forty-five to sixty-four have some form of cardiovascular disease, and they tend to have outcomes even worse than men's. Women are also ten times more likely to die from heart disease than from breast cancer and from *all cancers combined*.

For the most part, men and women share the same risk factors for getting atherosclerosis and coronary heart disease. The one notable difference has to do with the role of hormones. Women tend to be somewhat protected from heart disease until they become postmenopausal, when their risk shoots up to the same level as men's. Women as well as men need to focus on the basics and live a heart-healthy lifestyle to prevent coronary heart disease.

Summing It Up

Coronary heart disease is a leading killer of both men and women throughout the world. Atherosclerosis, the underlying cause of coronary heart disease and heart attacks, is a complex inflammatory reaction that damages arteries throughout the body.

Thanks to sedentary lifestyles and the fat-laden American diet, atherosclerosis now commonly begins in kids as young as twelve and thirteen years old. Atherosclerosis is sparked by risk factors such as smoking, obesity, high blood pressure, high bad cholesterol, and low good cholesterol.

Take charge of your life by taking charge of your arteries. Make heart health a priority, and keep your heart defenses strong—preventing heart disease is the best form of treatment. Also take advantage of the newest ways to detect endothelial dysfunction, coronary artery inflammation, and cholesterol plaque formation (see Step Three of this program). All of these detection methods will give you the best chance of beating this deadly disease.

STEP TWO

Take Charge of Your Cardiac Risk Factors

S tep One of the Heart Smart Program gave you the tools you need to recognize the warning signs and symptoms of a heart attack and other life-threatening causes of chest pain. It also introduced you to atherosclerosis, the underlying process that causes coronary heart disease.

Now it's time to shift gears.

It's time to start targeting your risk *for coronary heart disease.*

Step Two starts you down the path of a proven and easy-to-follow process that will help you prevent or defeat the destructive and deadly effects of coronary heart disease. You may be shocked to learn that physicians are not adequately screening for and treating coronary heart disease risk factors in seven out of ten of their patients. It is a big mistake to assume that you have been adequately screened for coronary heart disease.

In this section I provide an overview and capsule summary of all the "traditional" cardiac risk factors before taking an in-depth look at the "big five" killers: high blood pressure, the "new" diabetes, smoking, obesity, and a sedentary lifestyle.

Finally we'll get to the term that most of us are familiar with when it comes to heart disease: cholesterol. You'll learn what causes your cholesterol to get out of whack and get a detailed Heart Smart plan to lower your bad cholesterol, lower your triglycerides, and raise your good cholesterol levels.

You Need to Know Your Cardiac Risk Factors

Once you understand your risks for coronary heart disease, you can

- *Prevent* coronary heart disease from ever developing
- *Reverse* coronary heart disease if you already have it
- *Eliminate* your chances of dying suddenly and unexpectedly from a sudden heart attack

Chapter 4

Traditional Cardiac Risk Factors
The Big Picture

To take charge of your cardiac risk factors, you first have to know what they are and how they affect you.

You mean my doctor doesn't have my risk factors covered?

That's right. Nothing against your doctor, it's just that the health care system has changed. Managed-care issues, decreasing fee reimbursements, and the need for your doctor to see more and more patients each day are realities of health care today.

Study after study has shown that doctors drop the ball when it comes to evaluating and treating your cardiac risk factors. *More than 70 percent of patients are not receiving adequate screening and treatment for their cardiac risk factors*, so make no assumptions about your cardiac risk.

- Don't assume you are at low risk for heart disease until you have had all of your cardiac risk factors tested and evaluated.

- Don't assume your doctor knows your cardiac risk.

- Don't assume your doctor is up to date on the newest prevention guidelines.

- Don't assume that because your doctor hasn't discussed weight, dietary, and exercise issues with you that they're not important.

- Don't assume that just because you are taking medication for high blood pressure, high cholesterol, or diabetes that you are at lower risk for coronary heart disease. You need to reach and maintain your target goals to lower your cardiac risk.

Much of the burden of protecting yourself from heart disease rests on your own shoulders. No one will put a higher priority on your heart health than you. By taking responsibility for your heart health you can and will prevent coronary heart disease and heart attacks. The facts that an American has a heart attack every twenty seconds and that heart disease is still the leading killer in the United States are all the proof you need that waiting for your doctor to take charge of your heart health is all too often a losing strategy.

Framingham Changed Everything

It's impossible to talk about cardiac risk factors without at least mentioning the Framingham Heart Study. It's because of this important study that we even have the term "risk factors." The study revolutionized the way we view coronary heart disease.

The Framingham Heart Study has been tracking and documenting the heart health of the residents of Framingham, Massachusetts, since 1948. Before the study began, atherosclerosis was believed to be an inevitable part of the aging process. Framingham debunked that theory and, over the years, has proven that underlying conditions (including diabetes and high blood pressure) as well as lifestyle issues (such as obesity and smoking) are directly related to the development of coronary heart disease. Data from the Framingham study also identified LDL cholesterol as a central player in atherosclerosis and showed the heart-protective effects of high HDL cholesterol levels.

The Framingham study is now turning its attention to the genetics of heart disease, and will likely open many new doors to the underlying mechanisms of coronary heart disease.

Are You at Risk? Don't Be Fooled

How do you know if you are at risk for a heart attack? You may be thin, you may exercise regularly, and you may even have normal cholesterol levels, so you may think you're not at risk. But is that really the case?

David thought he knew his cardiac risk. He was forty-three years old, thin, and played vigorous games of rugby two or three times a week. David was in great shape and had no symptoms, so he assumed that he was at very low risk for heart disease. He never bothered to actually test for any cardiac risk factors.

David started having left shoulder pain while he was running during his rugby games. The symptoms quickly progressed to the point that he would get shoulder pain with minimal exertion, such as taking the trash out. He was convinced that it was a shoulder injury but decided to check it out anyway.

David is now recovering from an angioplasty and stent surgery that opened the 99-percent-blocked artery that runs down the front of his heart. It turned out that David had two major risk factors—an extremely low HDL cholesterol level and high blood pressure—and had been at very high risk for heart disease for years.

Find out what *your* cardiac risk factors are before it's too late.

What Are the Traditional Cardiac Risk Factors?

Cardiac risk factors are traits or characteristics that help predict your chances of developing coronary heart disease. There are two categories of cardiac risk factors: traditional and emerging. We'll cover traditional factors here and emerging risk factors in chapter 7. The vast majority of people who develop coronary heart disease have at least one traditional cardiac risk factor: most have multiple traditional risk factors.

Some people, however, don't have any traditional factors. And even though that percentage of people is small, so many people have coronary heart disease that many of you will need to look beyond the traditional risk factors to the emerging factors to help determine your risk.

Ultimately, much of your risk for heart disease and heart attacks comes down to the choices you make every day. You can tackle coronary heart disease head on by recognizing your cardiac risk factors and aggressively treating them, or you can ignore your cardiac risk and come face to face with heart attacks, congestive heart failure, hospital procedures, bypass surgery, and even sudden cardiac death.

The good news is that it's *never too late* to figure out your risk for heart disease and heart attacks. If you don't already know your cardiovascular risk there is no reason to put it off any longer. Keep reading to learn about the risk assessment process that will help you prevent very preventable coronary heart disease.

New Findings on Cardiac Risk Factors

For decades most experts agreed that about half of all heart disease was caused by one of the traditional cardiac risk factors. The other half was a mystery. Many theories were put forth about what caused that other half, from genetic factors to yet undiscovered cardiac risk factors. But no one knew for sure what caused half the people who had coronary artery disease to develop it.

New light has now been shed on the subject of cardiac risk factors. The 50–50 finding has been proven to be way *off base*. In August 2003, multiple new compelling clinical studies published in the *Journal of the American Medical Association* have proven that close to 90 percent of fatal coronary events are related to one or more of the traditional cardiac risk factors. Now 50–50 has officially been replaced by 90–10.

Traditional Cardiac Risk Factors

There are two types of traditional cardiac risk factors. You cannot control the following:

- Heredity (family history)
- Increasing age
- Gender

You can control the following:

- Elevated bad cholesterol
- Low good cholesterol
- High blood pressure
- The "new" diabetes
- Cigarette smoking
- Physical inactivity
- Obesity and being overweight
- Stress

Let's look at each factor now before we go into them in depth in later chapters.

Risk Factors You Can't Control

While cardiac risk factors such as age, gender, and family history are out of your direct control, they are still important to evaluate and can be used as motivating factors to help you stay in control of the risk factors you can control.

Heredity (Family History)

Genetic factors can be a good thing or a bad thing. Some people have a genetic blueprint that may increase their risk of cardiovascular disease, while others have one that can actually protect them from the disease. To find out your genetic blueprint and to help determine your cardiovascular risk, ask your parents or relatives about their heart history.

If you learn that your Uncle Joe had a heart attack at age forty or your mom underwent bypass surgery at age fifty-two, you can count family history as one of your cardiac risk factors. To consider family history a cardiac risk factor you need to have a male relative who had coronary heart disease before age fifty-five or a female relative whose coronary heart disease hit before age sixty-five.

Heart Smart Advice

As you look into your family's heart history, remember two important points. First, Grandpa lived in a different time with a different mindset. Your grandparents and even your parents and their doctors did not have the same knowledge about blood pressure, cholesterol, and smoking that we have today. They also didn't have access to the same powerful medications that we currently have.

Second, just because you have a family history of early coronary artery disease doesn't mean that you're doomed. Don't panic! Turn your family history into a motivating factor to be as heart healthy as you can and to keep your cardiac risk low.

Increasing Age

If you're a man over age forty-five or a woman over age fifty-five, you have at least one risk factor for coronary heart disease. I haven't figured out how to slow the aging process yet, but living a heart-healthy lifestyle will make you feel ten years younger.

Gender

I don't particularly care for listing gender as a cardiac risk factor. Being male is often thought of as a risk factor for coronary heart disease, and it's true that men tend to develop heart disease at a younger age than women. But noting that men develop heart disease younger than women do can give the false impression that women are somehow not at risk for the disease. So I list gender here to make women aware that they are *just as much at risk* for heart disease as men are.

Your level of risk depends on the number of cardiac risk factors you have. Whether you're a man or a woman, you need to determine your cardiac risk factors to help you determine your heart attack risk.

Risk Factors You Can Control

Most people with coronary heart disease have at least one, and often two or three, risk factors that are completely under their control. Weight control, exercise, and a Heart Smart diet are often all it takes to rein in these dangerous cardiac risk factors.

High Cholesterol

High cholesterol is one of the major causes of coronary heart disease. In fact, it is such a central character that it gets its very own chapter in this book.

The term "high cholesterol" actually covers a number of separate risk factors. LDL (bad) cholesterol greater than 100 mg/dL, triglycerides greater than 150 mg/dL, and HDL (good) cholesterol less than 40 mg/dL are all are considered independent risk factors for coronary heart disease.

Lowering your cholesterol can help save your life—it reduces your risk of dying from heart disease by up to 40 percent. Make sure you know all your cholesterol numbers, not just your total cholesterol. Because even if your total cholesterol level is normal it doesn't mean you are in the clear.

High Blood Pressure

A normal blood pressure is 120/80 mm Hg. High blood pressure (hypertension) of greater than 140/90 mm Hg not only substantially increases your risk for heart attacks but also puts you at high risk for developing heart failure and strokes. And if high blood pressure is combined with other cardiac risk factors it can be especially dangerous. Hypertension, however, typically does not cause any symptoms, so you need to have your pressure checked regularly to find out if it is too high.

The "New" Diabetes

Diabetes, a spectrum of metabolic disorders that range from a total lack of insulin production to high insulin production in the face of insulin resistance, plays havoc with the arteries all through your body and puts you at very high risk for developing coronary heart disease. A fasting blood glucose level greater than 100 mg/dL signifies prediabetes and greater than 125 mg/dL signifies diabetes.

I refer to it here as the "new" diabetes because of all the new information that has just become available on Type 2 diabetes and the metabolic syndrome and their strong association with coronary heart disease. Newly released cholesterol guidelines go so far as to rank diabetes at the top of the scale for heart attack risk.

If you have a family history of diabetes, are overweight, or have elevated triglyceride levels, you should be on high alert for diabetes.

Cigarette Smoking

Lighting up a cigarette is like sparking a fire for the development and progression of coronary heart disease. Smoking increases your chances of dying from heart disease by two to three times and doubles your risk of having a stroke.

Cigars, pipes, and secondhand smoke also increase your cardiac risk.

Physical Inactivity

Americans are taking laziness to a whole new level. Fewer than one in six adults in the United States exercise regularly. This increasingly sedentary lifestyle has contributed to epidemic proportions of obesity, higher cholesterol levels, and high blood pressure, all of which lead to an increased risk of coronary heart disease.

Obesity and Being Overweight

The more overweight you are, the higher your cardiac risk.

Obesity is a major contributor to coronary heart disease and all its risk factors. If you are overweight or obese you also are likely to not be eating a heart-healthy diet. You probably also are not exercising enough and have high cholesterol, high blood pressure, and/or diabetes.

Inactivity and obesity go hand in hand to contribute to Americans' progressive health problems.

Stress

I have yet to meet anyone with a completely stress-free life. But stress alone doesn't cause heart disease—it's how you cope with it that may significantly affect your risk for cardiovascular disease and heart attacks.

Uncontrolled stress leads to increased blood pressure, poor eating habits, lack of physical exercise, increased smoking, and weight gain. In other words, high levels of stress and its consequences increase your risk of heart disease.

Summing It Up

There is clear and overwhelming evidence that most cases of coronary heart disease are preventable. The causes of coronary artery disease are no longer a mystery; just about nine out of ten people diagnosed with coronary heart disease have one or more of the traditional cardiac risk factors.

Start your fight against heart disease by finding out how many cardiac risk factors you have. Work with your doctor and check into all the cardiac risk factors one by one. Don't forget that the cardiac risk factors— high blood pressure, high cholesterol, diabetes, obesity, sedentary lifestyle, and smoking—are far and away the greatest direct causes of coronary heart disease and heart attacks.

Chapter 5

Watch Out for the "Big Five" Killers

Hypertension, the "New" Diabetes, Smoking, Obesity, and a Sedentary Lifestyle

What are we doing to our bodies?

There are more than enough diseases and conditions to worry about that are totally out of our control without adding to them a whole new group of medical problems that are caused by our own actions (or inactions).

If you peel back the layers of cardiovascular disease, you will more than likely find one or more of the "Big Five" cardiac risk factors: hypertension, the "new" diabetes, smoking, obesity, and a sedentary lifestyle. All of these factors should be under our control.

Let's take a closer look at these dangerous factors.

Hypertension

High blood pressure is a condition that causes an elevated force of blood against the arteries throughout your body. Over time this high pressure damages blood vessels, leading to complications in the heart, brain, eyes, and kidneys. Like diabetes, hypertension is on the rise because many Americans are exercising less and less, have poor dietary habits, and are gaining weight. In addition, the newest blood pressure guidelines have lowered what is considered normal blood pressure, putting millions more Americans into the high-blood-pressure category.

A scary thing about high blood pressure is that it affects some of the "healthiest" people I know. People in top physical condition without an ounce of body fat can have high blood pressure. Certainly risk factors such as obesity and inactivity put you at greater risk for high blood pressure, but anyone can have it. Currently more than *fifty million* Americans have high blood pressure—that's about one out of every four adults.

Another scary thing about high blood pressure is that it's silent and stealthy. The damaging effects of high blood pressure sneak up on you because there are no early warning signs or symptoms.

Measuring Blood Pressure

There really is no good excuse for not knowing your blood pressure. Having your blood pressure checked is one of the easiest medical tests you will ever have. A blood pressure check is quick, cheap, and painless, and may just help save your life.

Once you've had your blood pressure taken several times, don't be alarmed if you find it tends to fluctuate. Blood pressure readings change from minute to minute and from day to day. The key to blood pressure measurement is to take a number of readings and look for an average systolic (top number) and diastolic (bottom number) blood pressure.

What Is the Optimal Blood Pressure?

The optimal blood pressure is less than 120/80 mm Hg. You have high blood pressure or hypertension if your blood pressure is more than 140/90 mm Hg or more than 130/85 mm Hg if you are a higher-risk patient with diabetes, heart failure, or kidney failure.

If, like some people, especially those over fifty, just your top number is elevated (this is known as isolated systolic hypertension), you still have high blood pressure and need to be treated. Both the systolic and the diastolic blood pressures are important and should be evaluated and treated equally.

Don't Wait Until You Have Symptoms

If you wait for symptoms of high blood pressure to develop, it will be too late. High blood pressure is called the "silent killer" because it rarely causes any symptoms before it severely damages the eyes, heart, kidneys, or brain.

Blood Pressure Classification

The Joint National Committee on the Prevention, Detection, Evaluation, and Treatment of High Blood Pressure, or JNC, sets the national guidelines for the classification, goals, and treatment of hypertension. Their most up-to-date report classifies blood pressure in four categories: normal, prehypertensive, Stage 1 hypertension, and Stage 2 hypertension.

Classification	Systolic BP (mm Hg)	Diastolic BP (mm Hg)
Normal	<120	and <80
Prehypertension	120–139	or 80–89
Stage 1 hypertension	140–159	or 90–99
Stage 2 hypertension	>=160	or ≥100

Headaches, blurry vision, palpitations, or light-headedness may be your warning symptoms of high blood pressure. If you experience any of these symptoms, be sure to have your blood pressure measured. Don't let a stroke, heart attack, or kidney failure be the way you find out that you have high blood pressure.

High Blood Pressure Complications

There is a direct correlation between the severity of high blood pressure and the risk of complications from high blood pressure: the higher the blood pressure, the greater the risk.

For the middle-aged adult, for every 20-mm Hg increase in systolic blood pressure or 10-mm Hg increase in diastolic blood pressure, the risk of cardiovascular complications doubles. That means that if your blood pressure is 155/75, you have double the risk of a heart attack than if your blood pressure were normal.

While it takes many years before significant complications from high blood pressure arise, having regular checks will tell you if your blood pressure may be a problem. Early detection and treatment can prevent all of the damaging effects of hypertension, which are

- Heart attack
- Stroke
- Heart failure
- Blindness
- Kidney failure
- Abnormal heart rhythms

Seven Steps to Blood Pressure Control

Well over half of the people with high blood pressure are not being treated aggressively enough. Simply being on a blood pressure medication does not necessarily mean that you are effectively being treated.

While your doctor will support and guide you, most people with high blood pressure need to take charge of their own treatment. Lifestyle changes, including losing weight, increasing exercise, limiting stress, and limiting salt intake, are key components of blood pressure treatment. If you can make these changes and stick with them, they may be all the treatment you require.

Make a serious commitment to your own health by making these important lifestyle changes. Treat early and continue treating until you reach your target blood pressure goals.

The seven steps to maximize your chances of bringing your blood pressure down to goal are: maintaining an ideal weight, following the DASH diet, following a low-salt diet, increasing your exercise level, limiting or eliminating alcohol intake, stopping smoking, and taking high-blood-pressure medications.

The ways to attack and lower your blood pressure are in your hands. Eating high-fat and salty foods, being obese, exercising infrequently, being highly stressed, and smoking all contribute to the development of hypertension. In fact, taken together these *completely preventable* high-blood-pressure risk factors account for three-quarters of all cases of hypertension.

The good news is that by making changes in your lifestyle, you may be able to partially or completely control high blood pressure. Let's take a closer look at the seven things you can do to lower your blood pressure.

Maintain an Ideal Weight

Lowering and controlling weight is a recurring theme throughout this book. Being overweight or obese is a major risk factor for developing

Hypertension Treatment Options

Treatment	Recommendation	Approximate SBP Reduction[‡]
Weight loss/ maintaining an ideal weight	Maintain normal body weight (18.5–24.9 BMI)	5–20 mm Hg for every 10 kg of weight loss
DASH* diet	Eat fruits, vegetables, and low-fat foods	8–14 mm Hg
Low-salt diet	Restrict sodium to 2.3 gm/day	2–8 mm Hg
Increasing physical activity	Exercise 45–60 min. 5 or more days/week	4–9 mm Hg
Limiting alcohol intake[†]	Limit men, 2 drinks/day; women, 1 drink/day	2–4 mm Hg
Stop smoking	Stop all forms of tobacco and nicotine forever!	5–15 mm Hg
BP-lowering medications	Use if unable to control BP with lifestyle changes	Variable (whatever it takes)

*DASH = Dietary Approaches to Stop Hypertension
[†]1 drink = 12 oz. beer, 4–5 oz. wine, or 1–2 oz. 80-proof spirits
[‡]SBP = systolic blood pressure

high blood pressure. Up to 75 percent of obese people have high blood pressure, though it's not yet entirely clear why obesity causes the condition.

One of the reasons appears to be that an enlarged abdomen activates hormones throughout the body that affect blood pressure, heart rate, and kidney function. Genetics also seems to play a role because some extremely obese people surprisingly maintain a normal blood pressure.

Losing weight, however, is generally a reliable and powerful way to lower blood pressure. Losing 20 pounds, for example, can lower systolic blood pressure by up to 7–10 mm Hg. Even minimal weight loss will help lower blood pressure and help prevent heart attacks and strokes.

Follow the DASH Diet

My patients always ask me if there is a diet they can follow that will help them lower their blood pressure. In fact, there is—it's called the DASH diet, which stands for Dietary Approaches to Stop Hypertension. In a major clinical trial the DASH diet was proven to lower blood pressure through a natural diuretic effect.

In the trial, patients who were randomized to the DASH diet excreted salt in greater amounts than those who followed a more traditional American diet, and had reduced blood pressure as well. The DASH diet lowered blood pressure by an average of 11 mmHg in patients with high blood pressure and even 3.5 mm Hg in patients with normal blood pressure. The effects of the diet were very similar to those produced by using commonly prescribed blood pressure medications called diuretics.

The DASH diet is a 2,000-calorie-a day diet featuring grains, vegetables, fruits, nuts, and low-fat dairy products. It is a well-balanced diet that is easy to manage with everyday items from the local grocery.

In addition to lowering blood pressure, the DASH diet is a very heart-healthy approach to nutrition and something you should consider even if you have normal blood pressure. Ask your doctor if the DASH diet might be right for you. For more information on the DASH diet, check out www.nhlbi.nih.gov.

The DASH Eating Plan

Food Group	Daily Servings
Grains and grain products	7–8
Vegetables	4–5
Fruits	4–5
Low-fat or fat-free dairy	2–3
Lean meats, poultry, and fish	2 or fewer
Nuts, seeds, and dry beans	4–5 per week
Fats and oils (good fats)	2–3
Sweets	5 per week

Follow a Low-Salt Diet

For many people, a high-salt diet may be a major contributing factor in the development of high blood pressure. Between work, taking care of the house, and going to the kids' soccer games, there is little time left to cook and eat home-prepared meals. Fast food, frozen food, and canned food make up a major portion of many Americans' diets these days. All of these types of food contain high levels of salt, for taste and for extended shelf life. Many processed and packaged food also contain high levels of hidden salt.

Salt (or sodium) is a vital component of normal cell structure and function and helps control the fluid balance in the body. The recommended amount of sodium for people with high blood pressure is less than 2,000 milligrams a day, but the average American eats two to three times that amount—a salty 4,000 to 6,000 milligrams a day.

A high-salt diet raises the sodium level in the body. As your sodium intake rises, your kidneys protect you by retaining extra water to balance out, or dilute, the salt. The more salt you eat, the more fluid you will retain; wherever salt goes, fluid follows. The excess fluid then builds up in the bloodstream and contributes to high blood pressure.

Restricting salt intake can bring blood pressure down by 2–8 mm Hg, or even more in particularly salt-sensitive hypertensive patients.

Increase Your Exercise Level

Regular physical exercise is a central part of staying healthy. Regular moderate-intensity exercise lowers your risk of high blood pressure by up to 50 percent compared to the risk of inactive couch potatoes.

Exercise isn't just good for high blood pressure; it also is good for the bones, maintaining or lowering your weight, lowering cholesterol, relieving stress, and reducing your risk of heart attacks. It also can be a lot of fun.

To be Heart Smart, I recommend that you exercise moderately five or six days a week for at least forty-five minutes a day. Any form of exercise that increases your heart rate (aerobic exercise) is great for blood pressure control and for general heart health. See chapter 12 for a complete Heart Smart guide to heart fitness.

Limit or Eliminate Alcohol Intake

While there may be some heart-healthy benefits to consuming small to moderate amounts of alcohol, the downsides of drinking too much alcohol must always be taken into account. In other words, too much of a good thing will hurt you.

Studies show that if you drink more than three alcoholic drinks daily, you are three times more likely to develop high blood pressure than someone who does not drink alcohol. Women who drink more than one and a half drinks a day have an increased risk of developing hypertension. Heavy alcohol use and binge drinking will markedly increase both men's and women's risk of high blood pressure and stroke.

On the plus side, at least one study showed that women who drink some alcohol but less than one and a half drinks per day have been found to have a 15 percent *lower* chance of developing high blood pressure. In addition, restricting intake of alcoholic beverages also can help you maintain or lose weight, since alcoholic drinks are loaded with calories.

Moderate drinking is defined as no more than two drinks daily for men and no more than one drink daily for women. An alcoholic drink is equivalent to either:

- One 12-ounce bottle of beer
- One 4- to 5-ounce glass of wine
- One or 2 ounces of 80-proof spirits

Be sure to consult your physician to see if the potential benefits from drinking alcohol outweigh the risks for you. If you are pregnant or have pancreatitis, liver disease, high triglyceride levels, or other serious conditions, drinking alcohol is especially dangerous.

Stop Smoking

The nicotine in cigarettes and other tobacco products causes your heart to beat faster and work harder. In addition, nicotine also causes a rise in your blood pressure. The blood pressure can rise 5 to 15 mm Hg with each cigarette. Whether you smoke two cigarettes a day or two packs a day, you are putting undue stress on your arteries, markedly increasing your risk of heart attack and stroke.

Smoking cessation will have an immediate and dramatic effect on lowering your blood pressure. Your arteries will be forever grateful the day they no longer are being constricted by nicotine and simultaneously hammered by high blood pressure.

Taking High-Blood-Pressure Medications

Blood pressure medications really work at lowering your pressure, and today we have some pretty amazing drugs to choose from. If the time comes that you need medication, your doctor will choose from hundreds available to find one that lowers your blood pressure safely, has proven benefits, and has minimal side effects.

The ideal blood pressure medication

- Lowers blood pressure to your target pressure
- Causes no/minimal side effects
- If needed, will treat other conditions you may have, such as heart failure, coronary artery disease, or diabetes
- Is proven to reduce the deadly complications of hypertension

Even with the ideal medication, beginning to take it can be a frustrating experience. Most people are used to taking medications to make them feel better—an antihistamine to clear up that allergy, an antibiotic to wipe out that infection, an anti-inflammatory to ease up that knee pain. But you usually feel fine when you begin a blood pressure medication regimen, so you don't see a positive change.

Because of that, you may be annoyed if the medication causes irritating side effects. So it's important to keep in mind that the reason we want to lower your blood pressure to 120/80 mm Hg is that *that's the level proven to prevent heart attacks, strokes, and death*.

The Medication Merry-Go-Round

Try to remain patient during the trial-and-error phase of finding the blood pressure medication that is right for you. No single medication works for everyone. Expect it to take weeks, maybe even months, to find the right dose of the right combination of medicines that will lower your blood pressure with no side effects or only minimal side effects. Whether it's the first or the fifth medication you try that works for you, in the end you will be glad you took the time to find the right one.

Using a Home BP Monitor

If you find you have "white-coat hypertension"—your blood pressure reads high at the doctor's office, probably from nervousness, but is normal at home—you can invest in a home blood pressure monitor and take measurements at home on your own.

I strongly encourage everyone who has borderline or high blood pressure to make a small investment in a home blood pressure monitor. Nothing will make your doctor happier than your bringing in a nice record of your blood pressure readings taken at home. Checking your pressure and keeping a record will make your treatment go much smoother and you will ultimately have better blood pressure control.

The more accurate home BP monitors go around the arm rather than the finger or wrist. The automatic digital monitors are just fine. I recommend that you bring your home monitor to your doctor's office at least once to make sure it's accurate and that its readings correlate with the readings your doctor gets in his or her office.

Classes of Hypertension Medication

There are five major classes of medications that are used to treat high blood pressure, each of which lowers blood pressure through its own unique mechanism. You may very well end up taking a combination of blood pressure medications from multiple classes to reach your blood pressure goal.

Diuretics

Diuretics are known as "water pills" because they flush potentially dangerous extra salt and fluid from your vascular system through the kidneys, which causes increased urination. Along with salt and water, diuretics will also cause you to excrete potassium, so potassium supplements are commonly prescribed along with diuretics.

There are two main types of diuretics: loop diuretics and thiazide-type diuretics. Thiazide-type diuretics are often the first drug class prescribed to treat uncomplicated high blood pressure. Thiazide-type diuretics are inexpensive and safe. They have been proven to lower the risk of the complications of hypertension.

Beta-Blockers

Beta-blockers help control your blood pressure, slow your heart rate, and prevent heart arrhythmias. Your doctor may choose to use a beta-blocker to lower your blood pressure if you have an additional medical condition such as coronary artery disease, congestive heart failure, certain arrhythmias, or migraine headaches.

Calcium Channel Blockers

This type of medication lowers blood pressure by keeping calcium from entering into cells, which causes blood vessels to relax and lowers your blood pressure. Some calcium channel blockers also have an effect on the receptors in your heart and can be used to control cardiac arrhythmias (such as atrial fibrillation).

ACE Inhibitors

Angiotensin-converting enzyme (ACE) inhibitors lower blood pressure and promote blood vessel relaxation by preventing the hormone angiotensin II from causing your blood vessels to constrict. These drugs will likely be part of your blood pressure regimen if you also have congestive heart failure, had a heart attack in the past, or have diabetes.

Angiotensin Receptor Blockers

Angiotensin receptor blockers (ARBs) block the hormone angiotensin II from getting to the blood vessels. This forces the vessels to dilate, which lowers blood pressure.

ARBs are the newest class of medication for blood pressure treatment. They are extremely well tolerated by most patients and have a similar effect as the ACE inhibitors. Your doctor may choose an ARB to control your blood pressure if you have underlying congestive heart failure, had a prior heart attack, or have diabetes.

Combination Medications

Taking your blood pressure medication is crucial, so doctors are always looking for ways to make it easier for you to take your medication every day.

One way to make your life easier is for your doctor to prescribe a combination medication rather than several separate pills. The average person with high blood pressure requires up to three or four different medications to lower his or her blood pressure, so pharmaceutical companies recently began combining different classes of medications into one pill. If you find yourself on three or four different classes of medications you may want to ask your doctor if a combination tablet might be right for you.

Cardiovascular Benefits of Controlling Blood Pressure

- Lower your stroke risk by 35 to 40 percent.
- Reduce your heart attack rate by 25 to 30 percent.
- Reduce the risk of heart failure by more than 50 percent.

The most common medication class found in combination form is the diuretic. Diuretics are safe, cheap, proven, and effective. You will find diuretics mixed with every other class of hypertension medications.

The "New" Diabetes

Diabetes mellitus is a disease that damages both the big (macrovascular) and small (microvascular) arteries throughout your body—including the coronary arteries that supply blood to your heart. This makes diabetes another one of the major cardiovascular risk factors. It also often occurs hand in hand with multiple other cardiovascular risk factors, such as obesity, inactivity, hypertension, and high cholesterol.

The reason I'm calling it the "new" diabetes is that we now recognize diabetes as being a spectrum of metabolic problems related to lack of insulin and insulin resistance. In addition, all the new research shows a strong relationship between this disorder and high triglyceride levels, low HDL cholesterol levels, and coronary heart disease.

Diabetes Is a Serious Threat to Your Heart!

The "new" diabetes should really be thought of as two diseases: a metabolic disorder of high blood sugar (from low insulin levels or insulin resistance) and a metabolic disorder of the lipid and cardiovascular systems. It is a very dangerous condition for your heart.

Diabetes is on the rise. Thanks to the American diet and lifestyle, the incidence of diabetes is exploding in direct correlation to the growing obesity epidemic. Diabetes is a devastating disease and the sixth leading cause of death in the United States.

Currently diabetes affects an estimated seventeen million people in this country, but roughly six million of those people do not even recognize that they have the disease. To put six million people in perspective, think of the number as equivalent to the combined populations of San Francisco, Detroit, Dallas, Phoenix, and Philadelphia.

What Is Diabetes?

Diabetes is really a group or spectrum of disease processes caused by the body's inability to make insulin, its inability to use insulin properly, or both. The result of these inabilities is a disorder that leads to the abnormal metabolizing of sugars, proteins, and lipids. In simple terms, diabetes really creates havoc in your body.

Let's take a little closer look at what happens in the body of a person without diabetes. Food is broken down into sugars that provide cells with energy in order to function normally. Insulin, made in the pancreas, is the hormone required to convert the sugars into usable energy for the body. Your body may need to use the sugars immediately, or it may store them for use later.

If you have diabetes, you either don't make enough insulin or your body doesn't recognize the insulin you make. Without insulin, your blood sugar doesn't get converted into usable energy forms, and, whichever form of diabetes you have, you are stuck with elevated blood sugar. If left untreated, high blood sugar over time will cause extensive damage to the blood vessels and nerves throughout your body. To prevent this damage you need good control of your blood sugar level.

How Can You Tell if You Have Diabetes?

Could you be one of the six million undiagnosed diabetics?

Recognizing and diagnosing diabetes early is critical to helping prevent the complications of the disease. Even if you have no symptoms, make sure you have a diabetes screening blood test at least once a year.

Recognize the Symptoms

The symptoms of diabetes can be subtle, but you can easily recognize them if you know what to look for. Protect yourself by knowing the warning signs of diabetes:

- Frequent urination

- Extreme and excessive thirst

- Blurry vision

- Fatigue

- Unexpected or unexplained weight loss

Don't let one of the complications of diabetes be your diabetes wake-up call.

If you are obese, have high triglyceride levels, or have other risk factors for diabetes, then you should be on high alert for the disorder and have regular diabetes screening tests.

Types of Diabetes

The three major types of diabetes and diabetes-like conditions covered in this chapter are Type 1 diabetes, Type 2 diabetes, and the closely related metabolic syndrome.

Type 1 Diabetes

Type 1 diabetes starts in childhood and is due to a complete lack of insulin production. This is a very dangerous problem. Type 1 diabetics are totally dependent on daily insulin injections to stay alive.

The cause of Type 1 diabetes is unknown, although it is thought to be caused by a combination of autoimmune, genetic, and environmental factors. In Type 1 diabetes your body's own immune system attacks and destroys the insulin-producing cells in your pancreas. Without insulin, your cells cannot obtain the sugar and nutrients they need for energy, and essentially begin to starve. Blood sugar levels skyrocket, causing excessive urination, extreme thirst, dehydration, weight loss, and generalized weakness. Many Type 1 diabetics develop a severe form of advanced atherosclerosis and coronary heart disease at a very young age.

Type 2 Diabetes

Type 2 diabetes is much more common than Type 1 and is primarily responsible for the marked rise in the incidence of diabetes.

Type 2 diabetes is caused by either a lack of insulin production or (more commonly) the cells ignoring the insulin. This insulin resistance (rather than lack of insulin production) occurs when your body makes all the insulin you need and maybe even more than you need, but your insulin receptors ignore the insulin. The receptors are resistant to the insulin.

This process makes for a high insulin level, which promotes obesity because the excess sugars in the bloodstream are stored as fat. The high blood sugar level also promotes artery damage throughout the body. It's quite a powerful and damaging one-two punch. Insulin resistance can lead to many of the same complications as Type 1 diabetes.

The onset and causes of Type 2 diabetes, however, are completely different from those of Type 1 diabetes. While Type 1 starts early, Type 2 starts in mid-adulthood, usually at about age forty-five. And while Type 1 diabetes has no clear cause and is not linked to dietary or lifestyle factors, Type 2 diabetes has a number of well-defined risk factors: obesity; high-fat, high-carbohydrate diets; and physical inactivity are the major ones. Some ethnic groups, such as African Americans and Hispanics, also are at high risk.

The Metabolic Syndrome

Now that we have a name for it, I recognize someone with this threatening disorder just about every single day. It's not quite diabetes, but it's close and just as dangerous.

The metabolic syndrome is one of the hottest topics for those in the field of cardiac risk prevention and coronary artery disease. This syndrome is part of the spectrum of diseases associated with diabetes, elevated blood sugars, and insulin resistance, but you can have the metabolic syndrome without having elevated blood sugar levels. Often the syndrome morphs into Type 2 diabetes.

What causes the metabolic syndrome? The culprits include being overweight, being physically inactive, and following a high-carbohydrate diet. This means that the metabolic syndrome is entirely preventable.

Do You Have the Metabolic Syndrome?

The answer is yes if you have *three or more* of the following conditions:

- Abdominal obesity: for men, a waist circumference greater than 40 inches; for women, a waist circumference greater than 35 inches
- Low HDL cholesterol: for men, less than 40 mg/dL; for women, less than 50 mg/dL
- Elevated triglyceride levels, greater than 150 mg/dL
- High blood pressure: systolic, greater than 130 mm Hg; diastolic, greater than 85 mm Hg
- A fasting blood sugar level equal to or greater than 110 mg/dL

Being overweight and inactive, and following a diet high in carbohydrates has become the norm in this country. The metabolic syndrome is a direct consequence of the American lifestyle, a fact that must be recognized and reversed before the damaging effects of heart disease occur. Having any three of the particularly dangerous risk factors listed above puts you at very high risk for developing coronary artery disease and having heart attacks.

Diabetes and Heart Disease

The effect of high blood sugar on your heart arteries is devastating. Three out of four people with diabetes die from heart and vascular complications. In fact, the cardiac risks of diabetes are so high that diabetics have a three times greater chance of developing angina, having a heart attack, or succumbing to sudden cardiac death than people who don't have diabetes.

Many factors contribute to the high incidence of coronary heart disease in diabetics. Most important, diabetes causes low HDL levels, high triglyceride levels, increased clotting, and endothelial dysfunction. As you read earlier, these factors mixed together exponentially increase your odds of having severe coronary heart disease. To add to the problem, Type 2 diabetes almost always occurs in people who already have cardiac risk factors such as obesity, high blood pressure, a sedentary lifestyle, eating an unhealthy diet, and being a smoker.

The complications of diabetes are irreversible. Once the damage is done, there is no turning back the clock. The longer you go with undiagnosed or untreated high blood sugar levels, the higher your chances of developing one of diabetes' devastating complications.

Treating Diabetes for Life

New medications, scientific breakthroughs, and improved understanding of the importance of aggressive treatment have made a huge impact and extended the lives of millions of diabetic patients. Diabetes treatment is complex and well beyond the scope of this book.

I do, however, want to comment on some of the more important aspects of diabetes treatment, especially when it comes to protecting against the deadly cardiovascular effects of diabetes.

Treatment Options to Protect Your Heart

Aggressive control of blood sugar levels, hypertension, cholesterol levels, and weight are central aspects of diabetes treatment. Since cardiovascular complications are the primary cause of death of most diabetic patients, extra emphasis is put on all of these therapeutic options.

Blood Sugar Control

Keeping blood sugar levels in the normal range minimizes the amount of damage diabetes does to the arteries and nerves. Good blood sugar control requires a multipronged approach utilizing diet, exercise, oral medications, and possibly insulin. The hemoglobin A1c blood test best measures long-term blood sugar control. By maintaining your hemoglobin A1c level to under 7 percent you can reduce your risk of heart attack, stroke, and heart failure by up to 56 percent.

If your blood sugar cannot be maintained by diet and weight loss alone, then medications will be prescribed to lower your blood glucose levels. There are a growing number of good medication options today. The most exciting new class of drugs used to treat Type 2 diabetes is the thiozolidinediones, better known as TZDs. TZDs (commonly prescribed as Actos or Avandia) work by making cells more "sensitive," or receptive, to the insulin your body makes. (Remember, Type 2 diabetes is primarily a problem of *insulin resistance* rather than a lack of insulin.) The TZDs not only can prevent and treat Type 2 diabetes but also have a positive effect on cholesterol levels.

High Blood Pressure Control

High blood pressure is classified as 140/80 mm Hg in nondiabetics but drops to 130/80 mm Hg for people with diabetes. Blood pressure control cannot be overemphasized if you have diabetes—you drop your risk of death, heart failure, heart attacks, and vision problems by 15 to 56 percent.

Both diuretics and ACE inhibitors have proven beneficial effects, specifically in diabetic patients, and should be considered first when turning to medications to lower blood pressure. The ACE inhibitors lower your risk of heart attack, stroke, kidney failure, and death by 25 to 30 percent. The beneficial effects of ACE inhibitors are so overwhelming that, without specific contraindications, *all* diabetics should be taking one of them (no matter what the blood pressure measures).

Cholesterol Control

The National Cholesterol Education Program recommends that all patients with diabetes lower their LDL cholesterol level to below 100 mg/dL, *whether or not* they have documented heart disease. Lowering LDL cholesterol with the medications reduces the risk of developing cardiovascular disease and lowers the incidence of heart attacks, strokes, and death.

LDL cholesterol isn't the only cholesterol problem diabetics face; low HDL cholesterol and elevated triglyceride levels also are common confounding factors. Fibrates are a good choice for this problem because they lower triglyceride levels and help raise HDL cholesterol levels. Niacin also may be used—just be aware that it may have the unintended (and unwanted) side effect of raising blood sugar levels.

Blood Clotting Control

A big part of the problem with diabetes is that it causes your body to want to make clots. The "prothrombotic" state is a big contributor to heart attacks, strokes, and peripheral vascular problems. Smoking cessation and taking an aspirin a day are recommended to help lower your risks of these debilitating consequences of increased clotting.

Dietary and Weight Control

Much of Type 2 diabetes is preventable and/or treatable with aggressive lifestyle modifications. Dietary changes, weight control, and regular exercise are the most effective treatments for Type 2 diabetes, which is predominantly a disease of the sedentary and overweight. By making the needed changes, Type 2 diabetes is completely in your control.

One of the most important of those changes is following a low-carbohydrate, low-sugar diet. Diet plays a major role in controlling all forms of diabetes, and keeping your carbohydrate and sugar intake low is the most effective way to avoid out-of-control blood sugar levels. All dietary sugars cause significant and prolonged elevations of blood sugar.

Medications All Diabetics Must Consider

Most of the medications discussed above are critical to the modern-day approach to diabetes treatment. I always make sure all of my diabetic patients, regardless of blood pressure or cholesterol levels, are at least taking an aspirin a day to prevent clotting (also known as heart attacks and strokes), a statin to lower LDL cholesterol (and prevent heart attacks and strokes), and an ACE inhibitor to lower blood pressure as well as for kidney protection (and yes, to lower the risk of heart attack and strokes). These three types of medication are currently being considered for a diabetes "super pill" or "polypill" in which all three would be combined into one tablet!

This is just an overview of some of the major treatment options for diabetes management and cardiovascular protection. Make sure you go into much more detail with and learn about all the options from your doctor.

Smoking

Smoking is one of the major cardiovascular risk factors. It is the number-one cause of preventable, premature disability, disease, and death in the

United States and accounts for almost half a million deaths per year. But while it's hard for me to comprehend why people still choose to start smoking, I do understand why people have a hard time giving up smoking.

Addiction to nicotine is so severe that only about half of my patients who suffer heart attacks give up smoking after their attack. No matter how close to death they come, no matter how many of their vessels are bypassed during open-heart surgery, and no matter how often they promise me they will give up smoking, only about half pull it off for the long term.

Gerry is a classic example.

Gerry swore off cigarettes right after his emergency open-heart bypass surgery. Six weeks later he was smoking again. And nine months after that, Gerry had more chest pain, requiring an angioplasty and a coronary stent to open up another blocked heart artery. This time he really, really was ready to go cold turkey.

You would think that two major heart procedures would give Gerry some incentive to stop smoking. But at his last office visit I asked Gerry if he was still smoking, and he answered, "Not really." I thought I had asked a pretty straightforward "yes or no" question. But smokers never seem to want to answer it that way. "I've cut way back," "I smoke only on weekends," or "Not really," they say. Or they answer with my personal favorite, "Kind of." None of these is the answer I want, especially from someone like Gerry.

For Gerry, the fight—and the dangers—continue.

Four Excellent Reasons to Give Up Smoking

- One in five cardiovascular deaths is associated with smoking.
- The typical smoker is two to three times more likely than a nonsmoker to die of heart disease.
- Smoking doubles your risk of having a stroke.
- Smoking is a major cause of cancer, lung disease, and other medical conditions.

Nicotine Addiction

Nicotine is a drug, and an incredibly addictive one. Like my patient Gerry, smokers develop a dependency to nicotine just like many people do in other drug-dependent disorders. Nicotine stimulates the pleasure centers of your brain and causes both your blood pressure and your heart rate to rise immediately.

Nicotine's initial "rush" lasts about forty minutes. Then, as it wears off, your body starts craving more. This sets up a nasty cycle of nicotine stimulation, nicotine withdrawal, and then nicotine craving, which leads some smokers to smoke more than three packs of cigarettes a day.

Over time, however, nicotine's effect changes; it turns from being a stimulant to more of a relaxant. The calming effects it provides are the exact fix that people think they need when they start having the anxiety, restlessness, and agitation that come with nicotine withdrawal. This dangerous cycle then feeds on itself.

Smoking and Heart Disease

There is no doubt that smoking causes heart disease. The data from the Framingham Heart Study told us that, way back in 1960. The nicotine and carbon monoxide found in cigarettes do a lot of damage to your heart and blood vessels.

Smoking breaks down your initial line of defense against the attack of LDL cholesterol—it damages the inner lining of the arteries, the endothelium. The dysfunctional endothelium then becomes ground zero for coronary disease, triggering atherosclerosis.

In addition to damaging the endothelium, the toxins in cigarettes cause other harmful cardiovascular responses, ranging from increased heart rate and blood pressure to coronary artery spasm and arrhythmias.

The Harmful Cardiovascular Effects of Smoking

- Increases blood pressure
- Increases heart rate
- Increases the amount of work the heart has to do
- Platelets become activated and "sticky"
- Causes dangerous heart arrhythmias
- Decreases the blood's oxygen-carrying capacity
- Promotes heart-artery spasm
- Damages the inner lining (endothelium) of the arteries
- Decreases good cholesterol levels

But the harmful effects of smoking (and inhaling secondhand smoke) are not limited to the heart arteries. All the arteries of the body are damaged by smoking, leading to strokes, peripheral vascular disease, and erectile dysfunction.

And the bad news doesn't stop there.

Not only does smoking cause heart attacks, but smokers also have bigger heart attacks, *worse outcomes* with angioplasties, and *more complications* at the time of heart surgery than nonsmokers. Smoking is a lose-lose-lose-lose proposition.

Passive, or secondhand, smoke exposure also substantially increases your risk of heart disease. An estimated forty thousand people die of cardiovascular disease each year as a result of being exposed to secondhand cigarette smoke.

The Good News for Smokers

The good news for smokers is that they can quit—and quitting does make a difference.

Just one year after quitting, former smokers' risk of coronary heart disease drops by up to 50 percent! The risk for cancer and other tobacco-associated problems also drops immediately. It's never too late to stop smoking.

The Heart-Smart Smoking Solution

There is no easy way to end nicotine addiction. There is no magic bullet, only hard work and some rough days. Nicotine is so addictive that only about one in four smokers who try to quit does so on the first try. But not only will your heart thank you for stopping, but so will your lungs, brain, legs, sex life, breath, family, friends, coworkers, and wallet. They will all start to benefit the minute you stop smoking.

What is the most likely way to succeed? Once you have committed to stopping, your best bet for optimizing your chances of staying nicotine-free for the long term is to use a multidisciplinary approach. This means you need to use medication and get professional counseling.

Fear of gaining weight isn't an excuse. Many people tell me they don't want to quit smoking because they are afraid they will put on the pounds. As a cardiologist I can tell you that I would rather have you gain twenty pounds and be smoke-free than still be smoking at a lower weight. We can always deal with weight gain at a later date. Stopping smoking cannot wait, because it will never get any easier to quit, and continuing to smoke will remain extremely dangerous to your health.

In addition to taking medication and seeking professional help, you can also do the following to help you stop smoking now:

- Stay active.
- Avoid places and situations in which you used to smoke.
- Hang out with nonsmokers.
- Use healthy foods or snacks as oral substitutes.
- Avoid alcohol, bars, and other smoking triggers.
- Don't give up if you sneak one or two cigarettes; just come back even more determined.
- Tell all the people you know that you're quitting and seek their support.
- Think healthy: you will look better, breathe easier, have more energy, feel less confined, and be free of the mess and stench of smoking.

The Bottom Line

It's time to stop being a slave to your nicotine addiction. Not only is smoking dangerous to your health, but it usually comes with a handful of other cardiac risk factors as well. Take charge of your life and dump the nasty smoking habit. Each cigarette you smoke takes five minutes off your life. By quitting you will markedly decrease your chances of heart attacks, multiple types of cancer, and sudden death.

Obesity and a Sedentary Lifestyle

Being overweight or obese and following a sedentary lifestyle definitely take their toll on the cardiovascular system. Each condition is a major risk factor for developing high cholesterol, hypertension, Type 2 diabetes, the metabolic syndrome, and coronary heart disease, and they are all at the core of much of our current health problems.

In just one generation we Americans have managed to turn ourselves into one of the most overweight and out-of-shape people on Earth. We are a nation of extremists, glorifying paper-thin models and actresses while wallowing in adiposity. Our kids have replaced playing outdoors with playing video games and having home-cooked, healthy meals with eating fast food. We are fostering a culture of laziness and apathy that leads directly to obesity and cardiovascular disease.

What Is Obesity?

Obesity is a chronic debilitating condition in which the affected person is enormously overweight. Obesity affects almost 60 million Americans (more than 127 million are overweight); its prevalence in adults has more than doubled in the past twenty years, from 14 percent to 34 percent, and in children it has quadrupled in the past fifteen years. More than 30 percent of African American and Hispanic children are obese

Obesity has multiple causes; it is also difficult to treat and is one of the major reasons why high cholesterol, high blood pressure, and diabetes are on the rise. The consequences of obesity account for almost 10 percent of our nation's annual health-care expenditures, and each year an estimated 300,00 people die from obesity-related causes.

Are You Obese or Overweight?

There are three accepted methods for quantitatively assessing weight: body mass index (BMI), waist circumference, and waist-to-hip ratio.

Body Mass Index

Currently the most widespread formula for classifying weight is the body mass index (BMI). The BMI is not perfect, but it is a useful quantitative way to estimate your appropriate or ideal weight. The BMI is a formula based on your height and weight:

$$BMI = \text{weight (kilograms)} \div \text{height} \times \text{height (in meters)}$$

The BMI classifies weight into five categories:

Weight	BMI (kg/m2)	Obesity Class	Disease Risk
Underweight	<18.5		
Normal	18.5–24.9		
Overweight	25–29.9		High
Obesity	30–34.9	I	Very high
	35–39.9	II	Very high
Extreme Obesity	40+	III	Extremely high

Waist Circumference

A new study published in the *American Journal of Clinical Nutrition* in 2005 reports that waist circumference (a measurement taken by placing a measuring tape snugly around the waist) more closely correlates with heart disease risk than does BMI.

A waist circumference greater than 88 centimeters (34 to 35 inches) in women and greater than 102 centimeters (40 inches) in men carries a high risk of the metabolic syndrome and coronary heart disease. Your waist circumference also is a good indicator of abdominal fat, which is another predictor of heart disease risk.

Waist-to-Hip Ratio

Instead of measuring just your waist circumference, you can measure both your waist and your hips. A waist-to-hip ratio of greater than 0.85 in women and greater than 0.95 in men means that you are overweight and also puts you at increased risk for cardiovascular complications.

The Consequences of Obesity

Obesity has many dangerous cardiovascular and noncardiovascular consequences.

Cardiovascular Consequences of Obesity
- Heart failure
- Heart attacks
- High blood pressure
- Pulmonary hypertension
- Heart arrhythmias
- Heart valve malfunction
- High LDL cholesterol
- Low HDL cholesterol
- High triglyceride levels

Noncardiac Consequences of Obesity
- Diabetes
- The metabolic syndrome
- Sleep apnea

- Menstrual irregularities
- Depression
- Gallbladder disease
- Osteoarthritis
- Some cancers

Weight is not the only factor in the connections between obesity and cardiovascular disease and diabetes; body fat distribution also is an issue. If you have *central* fat distribution—your figure is apple-shaped—you are at much higher risk than if you have peripheral fat distribution—your figure is pear-shaped.

Weight Loss Really Makes You Healthier

Even losing a modest amount of weight will have beneficial effects for your heart. It will lower your blood pressure, lower your cholesterol, improve your blood sugar control, and lower your risk for heart attacks.

So think of weight loss as part of your prescribed medical treatment regimen. By losing weight as well as taking medications, you will significantly reduce your risk for coronary heart disease and all the coronary risk factors, particularly these three:

Cholesterol

Losing weight has a beneficial effect on all your cholesterol levels. Weight loss will lower your total cholesterol, LDL cholesterol, and triglyceride levels. It also will play a critical part in raising your HDL ("good") cholesterol.

Diabetes

Overweight and obesity are major contributors to diabetes mellitus and the metabolic syndrome. Losing weight plays a crucial role in preventing or reversing these diseases. Weight loss will decrease central obesity, improve insulin sensitivity, and lower blood sugar levels in people who have diabetes or the metabolic syndrome.

Hypertension

For every kilogram (2.2 pounds) of body weight you lose, your systolic blood pressure will be lowered by almost 2 mm Hg. A 5-kg weight loss will lower your blood pressure by 8 mm Hg. By simply losing weight, you may be able to say good-bye to your high-blood-pressure medications.

The Weight-Loss Plan

If you are like most of my patients, once you decide to lose weight, you want to have lost it all in a couple of weeks. But you won't be able to lose weight and keep it off by using a quick fix—a fad diet isn't the answer. You need to set both short- and long-term goals for losing weight, and you need to remember that weight loss is a battle for the long term. Your weight loss should come not from a diet but from a change in eating habits.

The National Heart, Lung, and Blood Institute's expert panel on obesity makes the following six recommendations for losing weight:

1. The initial goal of weight loss should be to reduce body weight by 10 percent.
2. Your initial weight-loss goal should be one to two pounds a month for six months; then you should reevaluate.
3. Reducing calories, not just fat, is the only way to lose weight.
4. A diet must create a 500 to 1,500 kcal/day deficit to achieve a weight loss of one to two pounds per week.
5. Moderate physical activity for at least 45 to 60 minutes at least five days a week needs to be part of every weight-loss program.
6. Following a reduced-calorie diet as well as engaging in physical activity are the best ways to produce weight loss, decrease abdominal fat, and increase cardiopulmonary fitness.

The Need for Physical Activity

Physical inactivity is a risk factor for heart disease, just as smoking, high blood pressure, and high cholesterol are. Physical inactivity leads to obesity, hypertension, high cholesterol, high blood sugar, weaker bones and joints, and general fatigue.

Regular physical activity plays a central role in good cardiovascular and general health. Exercise can help lower your weight, lower your blood pressure, and improve your cholesterol and blood sugar levels. You need regular moderate-intensity exercise to stay healthy.

But if you are like a lot of my patients, your day just gets gobbled up: a two-hour commute, perhaps as many as ten hours at the job, dinner with the family, putting the kids to bed, paying the bills, and a little R&R

before the whole cycle starts again. But no matter how tough it is, you need to make exercise a priority.

Right now there is an alarming trend toward physical inactivity that begins in childhood and carries over into adulthood. One in three teenagers reports no significant physical activity during the prior month. Three out of four adults report no physical activity over the prior *six* months.

What's your excuse for not exercising? The most common reason I hear is "I don't have enough time." If you need help in making exercise a priority—and an enjoyable part of a heart-healthy way of life—then turn to chapter 12 for tips and helpful information.

Summing It Up

Our bad habits are killing us. Smoking, obesity, and a sedentary lifestyle are major independent risk factors that directly contribute to coronary heart disease, hypertension, high LDL cholesterol, low LDL cholesterol, high triglyceride levels, and the "new" diabetes.

If you really want to prevent a heart attack and sudden cardiac death you must take a close look at your body, your habits, and your lifestyle. By taking charge of these controllable risk factors you can do more for your health than all of our tests, surgeries, and medications combined. Check out Step Five for more detailed information on starting a heart-healthy lifestyle that will help you start exercising and lose weight.

Chapter 6

Taking Aim at HDL, LDL, and Triglycerides

A New Look at Some Old Foes

The question today is no longer whether high cholesterol is bad for you; the question is how low your cholesterol should be. Clinical trials, scientific data from animals and humans, and cardiologists and expert medical professionals from all over the world keep coming to the same conclusion: *lower total and LDL cholesterol levels are always better than higher cholesterol levels.*

If you are hoping to read about "the great cholesterol myth" or want to hear about how the entire pharmaceutical industry and a few thousand doctors are involved in a giant conspiracy to trick you into taking cholesterol medications, then this is *definitely* the wrong book for you.

I am a traditionalist when it comes to cholesterol and coronary heart disease. I live and work in the trenches, which means I treat coronary heart disease every day, and I'm very familiar with the link between high cholesterol and heart disease. I have no connections to the pharmaceutical industry and I don't sit in a research lab all day. I do, however, believe in and use the latest clinical trials and expert guidelines relating to cholesterol and apply them to the care of patients every day.

There is no doubt that evaluating, detecting, and aggressively treating abnormal cholesterol levels lower your risk of coronary artery disease; peripheral vascular disease; heart surgeries; strokes; and, most important, death.

In this chapter I'm going to give you the critical information about cholesterol that your doctor might feel he or she doesn't have the time to tell you. First I will tell you a little about cholesterol in general and where it comes from. Then you will learn all about good cholesterol; bad cholesterol; and, finally, triglycerides. Each section will cover the subject in depth and provide the Heart Smart approach to fixing the problem. I'll also tell you how to get your cholesterol levels tested, when to get tested, what the tests mean, and how to treat abnormal levels.

As an added bonus—just for skeptics—I have included the results of some of the major groundbreaking clinical trials that prove that lowering your cholesterol will definitely benefit you.

So read on to find out if your cholesterol is something you should be concerned about.

Where Does Cholesterol Come From?

Your body has a love/hate relationship with cholesterol. Despite all you hear to the contrary, you actually *need* cholesterol. You just don't need nearly as much as you probably have.

Cholesterol is a soft, waxy, fatlike substance that is a normal and vital component of your cellular makeup and function.

So where does it come from?

Cholesterol comes from two sources: either your body makes it, or it's in some of the foods you eat.

1. Your body normally produces cholesterol (about 1,000 milligrams of it a day, to be exact). It is made in the liver and transported throughout the body in the bloodstream, attached to special transporters called lipoproteins. The 1,000 milligrams a day are all the cholesterol your body needs to maintain normal function.

2. Cholesterol also enters your body through some of the foods you eat, specifically the animal products you eat. Red meat, chicken, egg yolks, cheese, and milk are common foods that contain cholesterol. *Vegetables, fruits, grains, and other plant-based foods do not contain cholesterol.* Cholesterol comes only from animal sources.

It's Time to Get Tested

Being ignorant about your cholesterol levels will not keep you at low risk for heart problems. Cholesterol and coronary heart disease have no mercy on those who are "too busy" to have their levels checked.

Lower your risk by asking the important questions, first of yourself, then of your doctor: When was the last time I had my cholesterol checked? Do I know my good and bad cholesterol levels? How about that other thing I hear about, triglycerides? Do I have a protective cholesterol ratio or a dangerous cholesterol ratio?

If you've had your cholesterol levels checked recently and you can honestly answer all of these questions in a positive fashion, I applaud you. That is really great news. But if you can't answer all the questions positively or if you haven't had a recent cholesterol check, I suggest that you get the blood test done right away.

Taking the Test

The test for checking your cholesterol level is a simple blood test.

There is absolutely no way to know your risk for heart disease if you don't take the test and know your cholesterol levels.

The blood test is called a complete lipoprotein profile. It reports your total cholesterol, LDL cholesterol, HDL cholesterol, triglycerides, and a cholesterol ratio.

For the most accurate results, you need to fast—no eating or drinking—for at least twelve hours before taking the test (you may take any medications you need with a few sips of water). Your test results will be available within twenty-four to forty-eight hours.

Everyone over age twenty should have a blood test done to screen their cholesterol levels. If your cholesterol numbers are fantastic at age twenty and you have no other cardiac risk factors, you get a five-year pass (unless something changes during that time) until you should check them again. Once you hit the decrepit old age of thirty, you should have at least an annual fasting lipid panel done. But remember, these are all just guidelines, so use your common sense about when you should be tested.

What Does It All Mean?

Congratulations—you had a complete lipoprotein profile done, and now it's time to look at your results. When you read the results, you'll be looking at a lot of information. Here are the levels that will be provided.

Total Cholesterol

Your total cholesterol is the product of your good cholesterol, your bad cholesterol, your triglycerides, and a number of smaller, less-well-known lipoproteins such as the very-low-density lipoprotein (VLDL). The optimal total cholesterol level is less than 200 mg/dL.

All treatment guidelines emphasize your good and bad cholesterol levels as bases for prevention and treatment of coronary heart disease. A "normal" total cholesterol level may still leave you at high risk for heart disease.

LDL Cholesterol

Low-density lipoprotein, or LDL cholesterol, is the "bad" cholesterol. LDL is the primary source of your cholesterol and is your number-one target for heart disease prevention and treatment. The optimal LDL cholesterol level is less than 100 mg/dL.

Your LDL target is based on your overall risk for coronary heart disease. A level less than 100 mg/dL prevents atherosclerosis and may even reverse cholesterol buildup.

HDL Cholesterol

High-density lipoprotein, or HDL cholesterol, is the "good" cholesterol. It is the scavenger cholesterol that removes bad cholesterol from the arteries and takes it back to the liver for disposal. The optimal HDL cholesterol level is greater than 40 mg/dL.

While 40 mg/dL is the minimal optimal goal for HDL, this good cholesterol is so protective that you can really lower your heart disease risk by cranking your HDL level up as high as possible. HDL levels above 60 mg/dL are extremely protective for your heart.

Triglycerides

Triglycerides are another independent risk factor for coronary heart disease. Triglycerides are your body's storage form of fat. When triglycerides get broken down in the body they form remnants that can attack your heart arteries, just as bad LDL cholesterol can. Their level is part of every lipid panel and is commonly elevated if you have diabetes or the metabolic syndrome, follow a high-carbohydrate diet, or are obese. The optimal triglycerides level is less than 150 mg/dL.

Cholesterol Ratio

This ratio, which is the ratio of your HDL level to your total cholesterol level, helps to identify cardiac risk. If your cholesterol ratio is high, then you have an increased risk for coronary heart disease. The optimal cholesterol ratio is less than 3.5.

While the ratio may be interesting to know, all treatment guidelines are based on the absolute numbers of your good and bad cholesterol.

The Cholesterol Breakdown

All cholesterol, whether bad or good, travels in the bloodstream. Since cholesterol isn't capable of independent travel, it has to hitch a ride with special transport particles called lipoproteins, which are fat proteins.

There are three major lipoproteins: low-density lipoproteins (LDL), high-density lipoproteins (HDL), and triglyceride-rich lipoproteins (triglycerides).

We're going to look at each of them now, and I'll tell you what causes them to get out of control. Then we'll spend quite a bit of time focusing on the Heart Smart approach to getting your cholesterol levels back to normal and under your control.

LDL Cholesterol: Your Number-One Enemy

LDL cholesterol is your prime target and number-one enemy when it comes to predicting, preventing, and treating coronary heart disease.

Low-density lipoproteins are the major transport proteins for carrying around your cholesterol—they account for about 70 percent of your total blood cholesterol. LDL cholesterol is the primary culprit in the start of the life-threatening process of atherosclerosis, in which cholesterol invades your heart arteries. This is why LDL cholesterol is known as "bad" cholesterol.

LDL cholesterol and HDL cholesterol work on opposite ends of the spectrum. LDL cholesterol travels from the liver into the bloodstream and looks for weakness in your arteries' defense system. When it finds a weakness it attacks by invading the artery wall and setting up camp. HDL cholesterol, on the other hand, helps protect you by taking cholesterol out of your artery walls and delivering it back to the liver for disposal.

An estimated forty million Americans have elevated LDL cholesterol levels. If you're one of them, you want to start getting that number back into the normal range.

Great Reasons to Lower Your LDL Cholesterol

The benefits of lowering your LDL cholesterol are powerful, reproducible, and consistent no matter who you are. Whether you are young, old, black, white, rich, poor, a man, or a woman doesn't make a difference—everyone with high cholesterol benefits from lowering his or her cholesterol.

What happens when you bring your cholesterol level down? You prevent coronary heart disease if you don't already have it and you halt or reverse coronary artery disease if you do have it. Either way you win.

How Lowering Your LDL Cholesterol Helps

- Reduces the formation of new cholesterol plaques
- Halts progression of any current cholesterol plaques
- Causes regression of existing cholesterol plaques
- Stabilizes and prevents rupture of existing plaques
- Prevents heart attacks
- Prevents heart surgery (open-heart and angioplasty)
- Prevents strokes
- Reduces risk of dying from coronary heart disease

Every little bit that you bring down your cholesterol goes a long way to lower your risk of damage and death. Just a 10 percent decrease in your total cholesterol results in a 10 percent to 15 percent decrease in your risk of dying from heart disease. A 10 percent decrease in cholesterol also results in a 20 percent decrease in your risk of a heart attack.

Keep in mind that getting your LDL cholesterol down to your goal is just the means to an end. Preventing heart attacks and death is the real goal of treatment.

Determine Your LDL Target

Every time I turn around there are new data showing that lower LDL cholesterol levels are more protective than higher levels. But how low your particular LDL goal should be depends on your overall risk for coronary heart disease. The higher your risk, the lower you must target your LDL cholesterol.

The *optimal* LDL cholesterol level is less than 100 mg/dL. It is considered optimal because at or below that level the process of atherosclerosis virtually comes to a standstill.

LDL cholesterol levels between 100 and 129 mg/dL are classified as *near optimal*, but there is a risk at these levels that heart artery blockages can begin forming. At the *borderline high* levels of 130 to 159 mg/dL, the atherosclerosis process progresses at a rapid rate, and at *high* levels, above 160 mg/dL, the process is markedly accelerated. Above 189 mg/dL is considered *very high* and very dangerous.

This classification system was developed by the National Cholesterol Education Program (NCEP) and announced in a report called the Detection, Evaluation, and Treatment of High Blood Cholesterol in Adults. The report is also known as the Adult Treatment Program, or ATP for short. The system is taken from the most recently released set of comprehensive guidelines (ATP III).

Unlike with HDL cholesterol (greater than 40 mg/dL) and triglycerides (less than 150 mg/dL), which have fixed, common goals for everyone, the recommendations and goals for LDL cholesterol are very specific and individualized based on your overall cardiac risk. So the following Heart Smart information gives you optimal target LDL levels according to individual needs and conditions.

- Target your LDL to <70

By taking your cholesterol down to less than 70 mg/dL you can expect heart disease reversal. *If you have coronary heart disease or are at high risk for coronary heart disease, you should target your LDL cholesterol to this level.*

The National Cholesterol Education Program's LDL Cholesterol Classifications

Classification	LDL Cholesterol Level (mg/dL)
Superb: reverses coronary disease*	<70
Optimal: prevents coronary disease	<100
Near optimal	100–129
Borderline high	130–159
High	160–189
Very high	≥190

*Author's addition based on newest clinical trials.

- Target your LDL to <100

You can halt the progression of atherosclerosis if you keep your LDL to less than 100 mg/dL. *If you are at moderate risk for coronary heart disease, this is your target.* Many experts now suggest that everyone should target their LDL levels to *at least* this level.

- Target your LDL to <130

If you have one cardiac risk factor and are at low overall risk for coronary heart disease, this is your target. If your one cardiac risk factor is either smoking or diabetes, you should be more aggressive and target your LDL cholesterol to less than 100 mg/dL.

- Target your LDL to <160

If you have *no cardiac risk factors* and are at very low risk for coronary heart disease, we cut you a little slack with your goal LDL cholesterol level, with a target of less than 160 mg/dL.

How Did Your LDL Cholesterol Get So High?

If your cholesterol level is up there, most likely you have your eating habits and lifestyle choices to thank for it. But there are actually three ways that your cholesterol can rise to a dangerously high level.

1. *Your lifestyle promotes high cholesterol.* The vast majority of Americans have high cholesterol because of their dietary and lifestyle choices, all of which are contributing to the growing pandemic of high LDL cholesterol across this great (and increasingly heavy) country. The most common causes of high cholesterol are

   - High intake of saturated and trans fats
   - High intake of cholesterol-rich animal products
   - Obesity
   - A sedentary lifestyle
   - Smoking
   - Diabetes mellitus
   - Age (men over forty-five, women over fifty-five)

   All of these causes of high LDL cholesterol (except, of course, getting older) are 100 percent preventable and 100 percent under your control.

2. *Your body makes too much cholesterol.* A few of you may have genetic factors that cause your body to make too much cholesterol. A number of different cholesterol disorders can be inherited from your parents in the form of an overactive cholesterol-producing gene. A genetic predisposition accounts for a relatively small percentage of high-cholesterol problems in the United States, but be on high alert if you have relatives who developed high cholesterol at a very early age.

3. *You have a defective cholesterol sweeper.* Not only does your liver make and secrete LDL cholesterol, but it also helps remove LDL cholesterol from your blood. Your liver has LDL *receptors* that sweep LDL cholesterol out of your blood and dispose of it. If you have a lot of LDL receptors, your blood LDL cholesterol will therefore be low, but if you have a deficiency of LDL receptors, your LDL cholesterol will be elevated. Both genetic and dietary factors play a role in how many receptors you have and how effective they are.

The Heart Smart Guide to Lowering LDL Cholesterol

If you read the previous part of this chapter carefully, you now know what LDL cholesterol is, how to test for it, what causes elevated levels, your target LDL cholesterol level, and the overwhelming benefits of lowering LDL cholesterol.

That leads us to an all-important question, "Now how do I lower my LDL cholesterol?" The exciting news is that you can knock the heck out

---

Top Ten Ways to Lower Your LDL Cholesterol

1. Cut out the bad fats (trans and saturated fats).
2. Increase the good fats (monounsaturated and polyunsaturated).
3. Stick with low-cholesterol or cholesterol-free foods.
4. Maintain an ideal body weight.
5. Have no tolerance for smoking.
6. Control your blood sugar.
7. Start a regular exercise program.
8. Take advantage of cholesterol-lowering superfoods.
9. Go to the statin drugs early.
10. Consider using other cholesterol-lowering drugs.

of LDL cholesterol levels: on your own, and with the help of cholesterol-lowering medications.

You can see from the list that making changes in unhealthy dietary and lifestyle habits can take care of virtually all the reversible causes of high LDL cholesterol. You need to eliminate the bad fats and cholesterol from your diet, increase the amount of exercise you get, lose the extra weight, and stop the smoking.

Easier said than done, I realize. So the next part of this chapter focuses on ten major Heart Smart ways to make the needed diet and lifestyle changes. (Also see Step Five of the Heart Smart Program.)

1. Cut Out the Bad Fats (Trans and Saturated Fats)

My Heart Smart cholesterol-lowering plan encourages you to eat fat—but the right kind of fat. Eating the right kind of fat, the good fat, actually *improves* your heart health.

Eating bad fats, on the other hand, is basically like spoon-feeding LDL cholesterol right into your heart arteries. Bad fats are the largest contributors to high LDL cholesterol levels and coronary heart disease.

What are the good fats, and what are the bad fats? The major fats we eat are saturated, trans, monounsaturated, and polyunsaturated fats. Saturated and trans fats raise LDL cholesterol and increase your risk for coronary heart disease—they're the bad fats. Monounsaturated and polyunsaturated fats may decrease your risk for coronary heart disease—they're the good fats.

To stay heart healthy, you need to limit your intake of bad fats:

- Limit trans fats to less than 1 percent of your total daily calories.

- Limit saturated fats to less than 7 percent of your total daily calories.

- Limit all fats to less than 25 to 30 percent of your total daily calories.

The recommended total daily intake of all fats (good and bad) is 25 to 30 percent of total calories. Considering the average American gets about 30 percent of his or her daily calories from *saturated fats alone*, you can see that we have a lot of room for a healthy improvement.

What are saturated fats, and in what foods are they found? Saturated fats have all the hydrogen the carbon atoms can hold. Saturated fats are solid at room temperature and are the primary dietary cause of elevated LDL cholesterol levels. Saturated fats are found in animal products, including fatty meats, whole milk, ice cream, cheese, and butter, and in some vegetable oils, such as coconut, palm, and palm kernel.

Trans fats are the result of a process called hydrogenation (adding hydrogen to vegetable oil). These fats form when liquid oils are made into solid fats such as shortening or margarine. Trans fats are considered particularly dangerous because they not only elevate bad cholesterol but also lower good cholesterol; they are largely accountable for the current epidemic of obesity and elevated cholesterol in children, adolescents, and adults. In addition to shortening and margarine, trans fats are in many of the foods you and your kids eat daily, such as fried foods, processed foods, and commercially baked goods (crackers, cookies, muffins, doughnuts).

When you're shopping for groceries, try to avoid buying foods with labels containing the words "hydrogenated," "partially hydrogenated," "trans fatty acids," or "trans fat." These are all essentially code words for the fact that the product is full of a dangerous type of fat that, if not limited, will cause obesity and high cholesterol.

Making the dietary transition from eating lots of bad fats to eating a moderate amount of good fats is a critical step in preventing heart disease and lowering bad cholesterol.

2. Increase the Good Fats (Monounsaturated and Polyunsaturated)

Good fats eaten in moderation can actually lower your risk of heart disease by lowering LDL cholesterol levels, lowering triglyceride levels, and raising your good HDL cholesterol.

Two-thirds of your daily fat intake should be from one of the unsaturated fats, either monounsaturated or polyunsaturated. Monounsaturated fats include olive and canola oils; polyunsaturated fats include safflower, corn, soybean, and sunflower oils. Oily fish and nuts also are great and healthy sources of polyunsaturated fats.

All fats are high in calories, however, so even the good fats must be kept to a minimum.

3. Stick with Low-Cholesterol or Cholesterol-Free Foods

Many of the foods that are high in saturated and trans fats are also high in cholesterol. Dietary cholesterol comes from animal sources such as meat, poultry, higher-fat milk products, and egg yolks. Like diets high in saturated and trans fats, diets high in cholesterol also raise the bad LDL cholesterol levels.

To prevent heart disease and heart attacks, your daily intake of cholesterol should be less than 200 to 300 mg.

To keep your intake under that amount you'll need to turn to non-animal foods and look for products that are labeled "cholesterol-free" (less than 2 mg cholesterol and 2 gm or less of saturated fat per serving) or "low cholesterol" (20 mg of cholesterol or less).

4. Maintain an Ideal Body Weight

A waist circumference of greater than forty inches in men and over thirty-five inches in women increases your risk of high LDL cholesterol and coronary heart disease. Being overweight or obese is another leading cause of high triglycerides and high LDL cholesterol as well as low HDL cholesterol levels. Not only does obesity (mainly central obesity) cause increased LDL cholesterol levels, it also causes your LDL cholesterol to be the more dangerous *small and dense type* (see chapter 7).

Eating for comfort only, eating portions that are too large, eating foods high in calories and fat, eating too many carbohydrates and simple sugars, and lack of exercise all increase your risk of being overweight and having high LDL cholesterol levels. Being overweight or obese is not just an eating problem; it's also a sedentary lifestyle problem.

While trying to maintain an ideal weight should be your goal, any weight loss helps. If you are overweight, losing as little as 5 to 10 percent of your weight can make a big difference in your cholesterol levels and lower your risk of a heart attack. Make weight loss a priority for a healthy heart.

5. Have No Tolerance for Smoking

The nicotine and other carcinogens from smoke damage your arteries and alter your LDL cholesterol shape and size, making it even more dangerous. These changes promote buildup of cholesterol deposits inside your heart arteries, increasing your risk for a heart attack.

Smoking cessation lowers your LDL cholesterol, increases your HDL cholesterol, and drops your risk of a heart attack by 50 percent in the first year.

6. Control Your Blood Sugar

Diabetes is primarily associated with low HDL cholesterol and high triglyceride levels; however, many diabetics, especially Type 2 diabetics, and those with prediabetes or the metabolic syndrome, also have elevated LDL cholesterol levels.

The dangerous combination of high LDL cholesterol, low HDL cholesterol, and high triglycerides puts diabetic patients at very high risk for coronary heart disease—at such high risk, in fact, that the newest national guidelines suggest diabetics pay special attention to their cholesterol levels and aim for an LDL cholesterol of less than 100 mg/dL.

7. Start a Regular Exercise Program

Put exercise at the top of your list for a heart-healthy life. Exercise will help you lose weight, prevent diabetes, raise your HDL cholesterol, lower your triglyceride levels and lower your LDL cholesterol. If that's not enough, exercise helps relieve stress and makes you look better and feel better about yourself.

Just as with cholesterol-lowering medications, think of exercise as a prescribed treatment for protecting your heart. For optimal health, begin moderate-intensity exercise forty-five to sixty minutes a day for five or more days a week (see chapter 12).

8. Take Advantage of Cholesterol-Lowering Superfoods

Cutting out the bad fats and cholesterol is part of the LDL cholesterol-lowering equation; just make sure that in their place you add heart-healthy foods. Avocados, almonds, oat bran, barley, beans, legumes, flax seed, olive oil, garlic, and tofu are all foods that can lower your LDL cholesterol and lower your overall cardiovascular risk. More detailed information on all of these foods is given in chapter 13.

Nuts Nuts are high in fat, but it's the good monounsaturated and polyunsaturated fats. Multiple clinical trials have found that eating five to seven servings of nuts a week will lower your LDL cholesterol and lower your cardiac risk.

Nuts are high in calories, so remember that just a little bit of nuts goes a long way. Add a few tablespoonfuls of hazelnuts, almonds, pecans, cashews, walnuts, or macadamia nuts to your diet each day.

Soy The FDA recently approved the health claim for soy on its effects of lowering the risk of heart disease. Soy has been shown to reduce cholesterol levels by up to 25 percent in people with high cholesterol levels. To maximize the cholesterol-lowering effects of soy you need to eat at least four servings of 6.25 grams of soy protein, or 25 grams total, a day.

Soy protein is found in soy beverages and energy bars (probably your single best source of soy, containing up to 20 grams), tofu, tempeh, miso, soymilk, soy patties, soybeans, and soy powder.

Fiber Think of fiber as carbohydrates that can't be digested. Fiber is present in fruits, vegetables, grains, and legumes. Soluble fiber (fiber that partially dissolves in water) can help lower LDL cholesterol levels and lower your risk of coronary heart disease.

Oatmeal, oat bran, nuts, seeds, beans, lentils, apples, pears, and strawberries are all excellent sources of soluble fiber.

Eating the recommended 20 to 35 grams of fiber a day can reduce your risk of heart disease by up to 40 percent.

Fruits and vegetables Eating plenty of fruits and vegetables not only helps you lower your LDL cholesterol but also helps you lower your blood pressure, prevent strokes, lower your risk of some cancers, and guard against visual loss from cataracts and macular degeneration.

While all fruits and vegetables are beneficial to heart health, green leafy vegetables such as spinach and lettuce; cruciferous vegetables such as broccoli, cabbage, and Brussels sprouts; and fruits such as grapefruits and oranges are considered especially heart-healthy foods.

A Harvard-based study found that people who averaged eight or more servings a day of fruit and vegetables were 30 percent less likely to have a heart attack or stroke compared to those who ate less than two servings a day. Even if you can't make it to eight servings a day, for each extra serving of fruits and vegetables added to your diet a day you can drop your risk of heart disease by 4 percent.

Stanols/sterols Sterols are a subgroup of natural steroids found in plants. Their structure is almost identical to that of cholesterol. Stanols are a derivative of sterols.

Sterols and stanols have been known to lower total and LDL cholesterol since the 1960s. In 1999 several companies began marketing margarine, salad dressings, and other products containing sterols and stanols to help reduce cholesterol levels.

Products such as Benecol margarine spreads and Benecol Smart Chews (made primarily from sitostanol derived from pine tree wood pulp) as well as Take Control margarine and salad dressings (made primarily from sitosterol from soybean oil) are readily available at most supermarkets. These products work by inhibiting cholesterol absorption in your gut from the food you eat. Stanols and sterols can reduce cholesterol levels by 10 to 12 percent when used as directed.

To see the maximum cholesterol-lowering benefits, the recommended daily intake of stanol esters is 3.4 grams a day. To get to this level you need about four servings a day—for example, four tablespoonfuls of the Benecol spread or two tablespoonfuls of the spread plus two Benecol Smart Chews a day.

Garlic I have traditionally been a skeptic of the cholesterol-lowering claims made by the proponents of garlic. New evidence now sways me to believe that garlic can modestly lower your total and LDL cholesterol levels.

A meta-analysis of thirty-six randomized clinical trials showed that various garlic preparations consistently led to small but significant reductions in cholesterol, from 11 to 24 mg/dL after just three to six months of use.

There are many different types and preparations of garlic supplements with widely variable amounts of allicin (the sulfur-containing component of garlic thought to be responsible for lowering cholesterol). It is unclear if supplements or fresh garlic have more of a cholesterol-lowering benefit. Since the cholesterol-lowering effects of garlic are relatively small and there are no trials to show that eating garlic saves lives, I recommend the liberal addition of fresh garlic to your diet three or four times a week but do not yet recommend the garlic supplements.

9. Go to the Statin Drugs Early

When diet and lifestyle changes are not enough to lower your LDL cholesterol level to your goal, you may have to use medications to help you get it down. The first-line medication class that doctors use to lower LDL cholesterol is the statins.

Statins are a class of medications known as HMG-CoA reductase inhibitors. HMG-CoA reductase is an enzyme that controls the rate of cholesterol production in the liver. Statins work by blocking this enzyme, which results in two positive effects:

1. The production of cholesterol is slowed down.
2. The liver's ability to remove bad cholesterol from the blood is increased.

Both of these changes lower cholesterol levels by up to a staggering 50 to 60 percent.

Though statins' main effect is lowering LDL cholesterol, they also mildly increase good HDL cholesterol and lower triglyceride levels. But statins have many beneficial effects above and beyond their amazing cholesterol-lowering ability. In fact, their most important effects appear to be outside of cholesterol lowering. Statins' many positive effects include lowering your risk of cardiovascular events, myocardial infarction, and death by

- Improving endothelial function
- Regressing the lipid core (see chapter 3)
- Stabilizing fibrous atherosclerotic plaque (statins are often known as "plaque stabilizers")

- Decreasing atherosclerotic inflammation
- Decreasing clot formation
- Promoting artery relaxation (vasodilation)

All of these benefits make statins a life-saving group of medications. They have been proven time and again to prevent the need for coronary procedures and prevent heart attacks and cardiac death. You can reduce your risk of dying from heart disease by about a third by taking a statin drug.

10. Consider Using Other Cholesterol-Lowering Drugs

Sometimes statins are either not enough to bring your LDL cholesterol down to goal or their use is limited because of side effects. In either case, a second cholesterol medication may be added to or substituted for a statin drug. Fortunately, there are a number of excellent LDL cholesterol-lowering alternatives, including Zetia, Vytorin, Advicor, and fibrates.

Zetia   Zetia, or ezetimibe, is a new cholesterol medication that lowers your cholesterol by inhibiting the amount of cholesterol you can absorb from your gut. Zetia has only mild LDL cholesterol-lowering abilities when used alone, but is quite powerful when used in combination with a statin drug.

Vytorin   Vytorin is a newer drug that combines a statin (simvastatin) with Zetia in one tablet to give an extra LDL cholesterol-lowering boost. Vytorin is an effective drug to use because it blocks cholesterol at both its sources: the liver, where it is made, and the gut, where it is absorbed from the cholesterol in your diet.

Advicor   Advicor is another newer cholesterol medication with a unique niche. Advicor is a combination tablet with a statin (lovastatin) and an extended-release form of niacin. Advicor is an ideal drug choice if you have the common cholesterol disorder of elevated LDL cholesterol along with a low HDL cholesterol level. The statin portion of the drug attacks LDL cholesterol, while the niacin portion brings up the HDL cholesterol level.

Fibrates   The fibrates, another class of cholesterol-lowering medications, are another good but secondary choice for lowering LDL cholesterol. Fibrates primarily lower triglycerides, but they also lower LDL cholesterol by 10 to 15 percent and raise HDL levels by 5 to 15 percent.

You Want Proof, You Got It!

Lowering LDL cholesterol with statin drugs is safe and prevents heart attacks and heart procedures. It also saves lives.

Numerous prospective, randomized controlled medical trials have proven the benefits of lowering LDL cholesterol for both primary and secondary heart disease prevention. (If you are trying to prevent the onset of coronary artery disease you are taking *primary prevention* steps. When you already know you have coronary heart disease and your goal is to prevent more heart attacks, more procedures, and death, you are taking *secondary prevention* steps.) Here are a few highlights of groundbreaking, landmark clinical trials that looked at the effects of lowering cholesterol.

Primary Prevention Trials/Studies

A number of large, randomized clinical trials and studies have proven the benefits of lowering cholesterol in people without documented coronary heart disease.

WOS-COPS (West of Scotland Coronary Prevention Study)   In this trial, which included men without any known coronary disease, patients were treated with a placebo or a statin for five years. Men in the statin arm of the trial had their bad, LDL cholesterol lowered by an average of 26 percent. This led to a reduction in heart disease deaths by a whopping 22 percent.

AFCAPS/TexCAPS (Air Force/Texas Coronary Atherosclerosis Prevention Study)   This study proved the benefits of cholesterol-lowering with a statin across the board, regardless of gender, age, history of diabetes, or smoking. AFCAPS/TexCAPS showed a 37 percent lower cardiac risk in treated patients compared to those who did not take a statin.

These studies and many others have shown time and time again that the benefits of LDL cholesterol lowering, even in low- to moderate-risk patients, markedly outweigh the small risks associated with statin drug therapy.

Secondary Prevention Trials/Studies

4S (Scandinavian Simvastatin Survival Study) trial   The 4S trial lowered total and LDL cholesterol levels in 4,444 people with known heart disease and high cholesterol levels. The group of patients who lowered their total cholesterol to less than 200 mg/dL had a 42 percent reduction in heart disease–related deaths over the following five years.

The 4S researchers projected that widespread cholesterol-lowering would cut the general public's risk of heart attacks by a third and the rate of heart procedures, such as bypass surgery, in half.

CARE (Cholesterol and Recurrent Events) trial   The CARE trial studied people with only mildly elevated cholesterol levels who had suffered heart attacks. This trial showed that men treated with a statin drug who lowered their LDL cholesterol level to less than 100 mg/dL had a 20 percent lower chance of another cardiovascular event (heart attack, heart procedure, heart-related death) than those patients who did not lower their cholesterol. Women fared even better, with a 46 percent lower chance.

This trial and many others consistently show that lowering LDL cholesterol causes a 20 to 50 percent reduction in heart procedures, such as bypass surgery and angioplasty, as well as heart attacks and heart-related deaths.

The Heart Protection Study   This well-designed clinical trial evaluated more than twenty thousand patients with high-risk coronary heart disease. Unlike the many dozens of trials before it that focused on cholesterol and heart disease, this trial treated all the patients with cholesterol-lowering drugs *no matter what their starting cholesterol level.* Prior trials had given drug treatment only to patients with very high cholesterol levels.

After five years the patients treated with the statin were compared to those who had not undergone cholesterol-lowering. Compared to the untreated people, the patients treated with the statin drug had a

- 12 percent lower risk of dying
- 38 percent lower risk of heart attacks
- 30 percent lower risk of interventional heart procedures (bypass or angioplasty)
- 25 percent lower risk of having a first stroke

In addition to gaining these significant benefits, no major adverse effects were found in the treated group. There was no evidence of an increase in cancer, lung disease, psychiatric disorders, or osteoporosis.

Neal White, M.D., director of the Cardiac Catheterization Laboratory at San Ramon Regional Medical Center in San Ramon, California, commented on the Heart Protection Study:

"This is the trial that radically changes the way we try to prevent coronary heart disease. The Heart Protection Study proves that all high-risk patients, regardless of starting cholesterol levels, benefit from cholesterol lowering. They don't just benefit a little bit either, it actually saves lives."

The bottom line is that lowering your LDL cholesterol may save your life. Any method you use for lowering it, either by making lifestyle and dietary changes or by taking cholesterol-lowering medications, provides a significant benefit.

Breakthrough Study Alert

The Heart Protection Study showed that cholesterol-lowering is highly beneficial, saves lives, is safe, and should be provided based on clinical risk of heart disease, not cholesterol levels alone.

HDL Cholesterol: Protecting Your Heart

About one out of every four people with coronary artery disease have normal total and LDL cholesterol levels and normal triglyceride levels. Their only cholesterol malfunction is a low HDL cholesterol level.

But HDL cholesterol is too often misunderstood, misdiagnosed, and mistreated. Even today too many patients and way too many doctors are not aggressive enough at detecting and treating low HDL cholesterol levels.

I think many doctors downplay treating HDL cholesterol because raising HDL cholesterol level is not nearly as easy as lowering LDL cholesterol level. Elevated LDL cholesterol can always be knocked down to size with the well-tolerated and safe statin medications. But we don't have that luxury with HDL cholesterol.

Raising HDL cholesterol can be a challenge. That's because it requires a combination of *education* and *dietary* and *lifestyle* changes to make it happen. HDL cholesterol doesn't change much through the use of statins; and the drugs that do raise it pose some challenging side effects.

So rather than spending time counseling patients on how making diet and lifestyle changes may improve HDL cholesterol levels, doctors tend to ignore them. And rather than taking an extra five minutes to tell you how to avoid the side effects from the most effective medications, they usually just throw you on a statin and hope for the best. Quick? Yes. Effective? Not even close.

To increase your HDL level, you need to become an HDL cholesterol expert—discover your HDL level and, if it's low, learn how to raise it to the right level. The following Heart Smart information will tell you everything you need to know to keep your HDL cholesterol levels as high as you can get them.

What Is HDL Cholesterol?

Just like LDL cholesterol, high-density lipoprotein (HDL) is a cholesterol-carrying protein. LDL cholesterol carries cholesterol from your liver to invade your arteries, sparking atherosclerosis. HDL cholesterol does the exact opposite. It takes cholesterol out of your arteries and delivers it back to your liver for ultimate disposal.

While LDL cholesterol works against you, HDL cholesterol works for you. That's why you want to have your HDL cholesterol level as high as possible.

High HDL Protects Your Heart

Clinical trials dating back to the mid-1970s have proven that *low* HDL cholesterol levels are strongly associated with coronary heart disease and heart attacks. HDL cholesterol levels are on average 25 percent *lower* in patients who had heart attacks compared to patients who don't have coronary disease.

Over the past twenty years, the heart-protective effects of high HDL cholesterol levels have also been proven. *Specifically, HDL levels above 60 mg/dL appear to significantly reduce the risk of a heart attack.*

HDL cholesterol promotes reverse cholesterol transport, a process that attacks LDL cholesterol at its core, inside the dangerous atherosclerotic plaque (see chapter 3). It protects your heart by

- Removing LDL cholesterol from the core of atherosclerotic plaque
- Transporting dangerous LDL cholesterol out of the arteries to the liver for disposal in bile acids
- Stabilizing unstable and vulnerable atherosclerotic plaque
- Promoting anti-inflammatory and antioxidant properties

If your HDL levels are too low, your reverse cholesterol transport system loses its effectiveness, allowing LDL cholesterol to run amok in your heart. Healthy, high levels of HDL cholesterol power your reverse cholesterol transport system into overdrive, knocking out any chance LDL cholesterol has of setting up shop in your heart arteries.

HDL Cholesterol Guidelines

The newest national guidelines for cholesterol treatment issued by the National Cholesterol Education Program put increased emphasis on the importance of treating low HDL cholesterol. If your HDL cholesterol is below 40 mg/dL you have a strongly positive risk factor for developing coronary heart disease.

An HDL level above 60 mg/dL is very protective against heart disease and can really be considered a negative cardiac risk factor. And the higher the level, the less likely you are to have coronary heart disease. There is no upper limit for HDL cholesterol, and any increase in your level is going to help you prevent heart disease complications.

HDL Cholesterol Classifications	
Classification	HDL Cholesterol Level (mg/dL)
High-risk HDL	<40
Low-risk HDL	>60

An increase of just 1 mg/dL of HDL cholesterol provides an amazing 2 to 3 percent reduction in coronary events.

For example, if you raised your HDL cholesterol level from 35 to 41 mg/dL your risk for having a heart attack or dying from heart disease would drop by a whopping 12 to 18 percent. Take the level up to 45 mg/dL and your risk will drop by 20 to 30 percent!

The bottom line for HDL cholesterol is that you need to raise it as high as you safely and reasonably can, with a minimal goal of 40 mg/dL.

Patel had a look of total disbelief on his face when I told him he was having a heart attack. His wife, who was holding the couple's one-year-old, was in shock as well. Patel was only thirty-three years old; having a heart attack was the last thing he thought he had to worry about. He was especially surprised because he had been told he had a normal cholesterol level about a year prior to his heart attack.

Patel did not know his good and bad cholesterol breakdown. In turns out that his total cholesterol was normal but not his good cholesterol. Patel's only cardiac risk factor was that he had a very low HDL cholesterol level of 31 mg/dL. •

Almost all of my youngest coronary heart disease patients (ages twenty-five to the mid-forties) have very low HDL cholesterol levels or elevated lipoprotein (a) levels (see chapter 7).

Rory and Phillip are two other men I treated during the past year who had advanced coronary heart disease at young ages. Rory's story is the more tragic. Rory was a rising star in the financial world. He had his first heart attack at age twenty-nine. Two years later he died suddenly from his second heart attack. His LDL cholesterol had been normal but his HDL had been a very low 28 mg/dL.

Phillip was a painter and a single father with a seven-year-old daughter. He needed open-heart bypass surgery at the ripe old age of thirty-eight. His total cholesterol was 148 mg/dL but his HDL had bottomed out at just 25 mg/dL.

While low HDL cholesterol has consistently been shown to be a strong and independent risk factor for coronary heart disease, high HDL cholesterol clearly protects your arteries from LDL cholesterol's damaging effects. In fact, *I almost never see heart attacks in people with really high HDL levels (above 60 mg/dL).*

What Causes Low HDL Cholesterol?

Many of the same factors that cause your LDL cholesterol to be high also cause your HDL cholesterol to be low. The good news is that all of these factors (aside from the less common "genetic only" factor) are completely preventable and controllable.

Lifestyle factors that contribute to a low HDL level include being overweight or obese, smoking, physical inactivity, and a high-carbohydrate diet (that is, a very, very low-fat diet).

The Link between HDL and Triglycerides

HDL cholesterol has a couple of very interesting relationships that you need to be aware of. One of them is that HDL cholesterol and triglycerides are strongly and *inversely* related to each other. This means that

---

Causes of Low HDL Cholesterol

- Obesity and overweight
- Physical inactivity
- Smoking
- High-carbohydrate diet
- High intake of simple sugars
- High triglyceride levels
- The metabolic syndrome
- Very, very low-fat diet
- Type 2 diabetes
- Genetic factors

high triglyceride levels are associated with low HDL levels. Because low HDL levels and high triglyceride levels are both independent risk factors for coronary artery disease, when the two problems occur together, as they often do, your risk for heart disease goes up significantly.

The Link between HDL and Diabetes

Low HDL cholesterol levels are also commonly associated with Type 2 diabetes and the metabolic syndrome. If you have a low HDL cholesterol level you should be on high alert for diabetes.

It's Time to Raise Your HDL Cholesterol Level

There are many things you can do on your own to elevate your HDL cholesterol level. Doing so will be extremely rewarding—it will mean that you are really making some heart-healthy lifestyle changes.

To bring up your HDL on your own, you'll need to make a personal commitment to improving your health. You'll also need to put into action some Heart Smart know-how. Making dietary changes, losing weight, and increasing your physical activity are at the core of the solution. Many of the same steps that lower LDL cholesterol also raise HDL cholesterol levels.

More detailed information on all steps is found in Step Five.

Top Ten Steps to Raise Your HDL Cholesterol

1. Get your weight under control.
2. Limit cholesterol and bad fats (saturated and trans).
3. Increase the good fats (monounsaturated and polyunsaturated).
4. Lower carbohydrate and simple sugar intake.
5. Start a regular exercise program.
6. Drink alcohol in moderation.
7. Stop smoking.
8. Look to HDL cholesterol-raising superfoods.
9. Try niacin drug therapy (prescription-strength).
10. Look to other HDL-raising medications.

1. Get Your Weight under Control

If you are overweight, losing some of that weight is the first critical step you should take to raise your HDL cholesterol.

Part of the reason why excess weight leads to low HDL levels is because obesity promotes high levels and increases activity of an enzyme called *hepatic lipase*. High levels of this enzyme drive down HDL cholesterol levels. Losing weight will decrease the activity of the hepatic lipase enzyme, which in turn will raise your HDL cholesterol.

The hepatic lipase–HDL cholesterol link is a fact of life—you can't get around it. So as long as you are carrying extra weight, your HDL cholesterol level is going to be driven down. If you're serious about preventing heart disease, you'll start taking off your surplus weight immediately. It takes as little as ten pounds of weight loss to see a rise in your HDL cholesterol level.

2. Limit Cholesterol and Bad Fats (Saturated and Trans)

The foods you eat play a huge role in determining your HDL cholesterol level. And strange as it may seem, a very low-fat (with no or little good fats) diet can actually increase your risk for low HDL cholesterol and coronary heart disease. Finding the *right balance* of the *right amount* and the *right kind* of fats is key to raising HDL cholesterol levels.

All saturated and trans fats are dangerous and lower HDL cholesterol. Excess saturated fats lower HDL cholesterol levels by decreasing the production of apolipoprotein A-1, a protein that is part of the HDL cholesterol particle. Decreasing saturated fats, therefore, increases the production of apolipoprotein A-1 and increases your HDL levels.

Keep your trans fat and saturated fat intake to less than 7 to 10 percent of your total daily calories. Keep your daily cholesterol intake to less than 200 to 300 mg a day.

3. Increase the Good Fats (Monounsaturated and Polyunsaturated)

Remember that you want to increase the amount of good fats in your diet—the monounsaturated and polyunsaturated fats. Increasing your intake of monounsaturated and polyunsaturated fats will promote the production of apolipoprotein A-1, which subsequently will increase your HDL cholesterol levels. Diets richer in the good fats also lower triglyceride levels, which again raises your HDL cholesterol levels. See chapter 13 for a more detailed discussion of good fats.

4. Lower Carbohydrate and Simple Sugar Intake

Watch out for those carbs! If you're like most Americans, your diet is about 70 percent carbohydrates and 30 percent saturated fats. Both of these factors contribute to low and dangerous HDL cholesterol levels.

High-carb diets cause your triglyceride levels to rise, and when they do, your HDL levels go the other direction: they drop.

By limiting foods such as potatoes, sugar, flour, and white rice, you limit significant blood sugar spikes commonly associated with lowering HDL cholesterol levels. Aim for a more balanced diet by limiting your carbohydrate intake to 30 percent of your daily calories.

5. Start a Regular Exercise Program

Let's face it: regular physical exercise is the cornerstone of a heart-healthy lifestyle. Moderate-intensity physical exertion for forty-five to sixty minutes a day at least five days a week is what you need to maintain a strong heart.

There's no question that regular exercise also helps you raise your HDL cholesterol level. In addition, it helps you lose weight and lowers triglyceride levels, both of which (as you just read) have a very strong effect on raising your HDL cholesterol.

There is no time to waste. Read chapter 12 to learn how to start your Heart Smart exercise program today.

6. Drink Alcohol in Moderation

For those who already drink, moderate alcohol intake—no more than two drinks per day for men and no more than one drink per day for women—often causes a significant rise in HDL cholesterol levels (the mechanism for this effect is not yet understood). Most people, however, dramatically overestimate the amount of alcohol needed to raise HDL cholesterol and produce other heart-healthy benefits, so be sure to read all about alcohol and its effects on your heart in chapter 13.

If you already drink alcohol and plan on continuing to do so, I am happy to share with you the consistently proven benefits alcohol provides the heart. I don't want you think that I'm advocating alcohol as a "treatment" for HDL cholesterol. **I never recommend alcohol to people who do not already drink.**

7. Stop Smoking

Smoking and low HDL cholesterol are a particularly dangerous combination.

First, the toxic chemicals in nicotine directly cause HDL cholesterol levels to drop. If that were not bad enough, both low HDL cholesterol levels and smoking damage your initial defense system—your endothelium shield—making it less able to fight against the advance and attack of LDL cholesterol, even at normal levels.

When you stop smoking, your endothelium is able to strengthen its defenses. This in turn leads to a dramatic improvement in your HDL cholesterol level, which strengthens your heart. One study showed that within just seven days of smoking cessation, HDL cholesterol levels rose by as much as 7 mg/dL (more than 20 percent)! Smoking cessation is probably the single best thing you can do to raise your HDL level and reduce your heart attack risk.

8. Look to HDL Cholesterol-Raising Superfoods

Many of the same heart-healthy foods that lower LDL cholesterol also can raise your HDL cholesterol level. Soy products, olive oil, nuts, lentils, beans, fibers such as oat bran, fish, and even orange juice have all been shown to have a positive effect on raising HDL cholesterol.

The key is to substitute monounsaturated and polyunsaturated fats, fruits, vegetables, legumes, nuts, and fiber for the excess simple sugars, bad saturated fats, and trans fats in your diet (see chapter 13).

9. Try Niacin Drug Therapy (Prescription-Strength)

While all cholesterol-lowering medications have some effect on HDL cholesterol, niacin is the go-to drug if you suffer from low HDL cholesterol. Niacin increases your HDL cholesterol level by an average of 15 to 40 percent at peak doses. The drug also is effective at both lowering triglycerides and lowering your LDL cholesterol by 20 to 40 percent.

For the best effect, combine niacin treatment with the dietary and lifestyle changes discussed above.

10. Look to Other HDL-Raising Medications

While niacin is the go-to drug for raising HDL, you may need to add a second or even third drug, including fibrates, in combination with niacin to help raise your HDL cholesterol level to greater than 40 mg/dL.

Advicor   Advicor, as mentioned in the LDL cholesterol treatment section, does have an effect on raising HDL cholesterol levels. Advicor is a combination tablet with a statin (lovastatin) and an extended-release form of niacin. Advicor is the ideal combination drug if you have the common cholesterol disorder of high LDL cholesterol and low HDL cholesterol levels.

Fibrates   The fibrates are another class of cholesterol-lowering medications that also can raise your HDL cholesterol levels. Fibrates are especially nice to use because they also powerfully target lowering triglycerides, which often helps raise HDL cholesterol levels. Fibrates are commonly used as the first drug of choice for raising HDL cholesterol in diabetics who commonly have the combination of high triglycerides and low HDL cholesterol.

The Future of HDL Treatment

Side effects, drug interactions, and relatively small increases of HDL cholesterol in patients have limited the drug treatment of low HDL cholesterol levels for years.

Now, however, breakthrough research has opened up new doors for treatment options as scientists learn more about the pathways, subclasses, and complex interactions of HDL cholesterol. Man-made HDL infusions and the synthesis of enzymes and proteins that improve reverse cholesterol transport are two of the exciting new treatments that are leading the way to expanding options for patients with low HDL cholesterol levels.

The future looks very bright for successfully treating low HDL cholesterol.

Triglycerides: The Last (but Not the Least) Part of Your Cholesterol Panel

High triglyceride levels have long been associated with peripheral vascular disease and heart disease, but trying to figure out the exact role triglycerides play in heart disease has been challenging. The problem is that high triglycerides go hand in hand with so many other cardiac risk factors, such as obesity, smoking, physical inactivity, and a high-fat diet. That's made it difficult to prove that high triglycerides *alone* cause heart disease.

Finally, after sorting through the results of hundreds of clinical trials, experts now agree that there is convincing data that prove that high triglycerides levels are, in fact, an independent risk factor for coronary heart disease and heart attacks.

What Are Triglycerides?

Triglycerides are a type of fatty acid that is an essential part of the process of storing extra calories to use as energy when your body needs it. When you eat more calories than you need, these excess calories are converted to triglycerides and transported to fat cells (or adipose tissue) that store the calories until your body converts them back into energy.

In caveman times this energy-storage function was a lifesaver. Cavemen didn't have the luxury (or maybe I should say the curse) of an endless supply of food. Their fat stores helped them maintain energy during lean times.

Today, our sedentary lifestyle and mass abundance of food, calories, and fat mean that we never need to call upon our fat packages of energy, so they just keep increasing in number. Americans continually make fat deposits in their adipose tissue but rarely need to make fat withdrawals. This is a direct cause of our obesity epidemic and the fattening of America.

Just how do we take triglycerides into our bodies? They are the main components of vegetable oil and animal fat. Once ingested, triglycerides are stripped down into fragments that travel in the bloodstream with very low-density lipoproteins (VLDLs) and intermediate-density lipoproteins (IDLs)—cousins of the bad LDL cholesterol and part of what makes high triglycerides so dangerous. Both VLDLs and IDLs act like LDL cholesterol, invading the blood vessels and promoting atherosclerosis.

Triglycerides Classification

The National Cholesterol Education Program's Adult Treatment Program (ATP III) has finally given triglycerides the respect they deserve. The newest cholesterol guidelines classify triglycerides as an important and independent predictor of coronary heart disease and recommend a new and aggressive set of lower triglyceride goals.

Normal triglyceride levels have been lowered from less than 200 mg/dL to the new level of less then 150 mg/dL. The standards for

New Triglycerides Classifications	
Classification	*Triglyceride Level (mg/dL)*
Normal	<150
Borderline high	150–199
High	200–499
Very high	≥500

borderline, high, and very high also have been lowered. According to the new guidelines, if your triglyceride level is above 150 mg/dL you have *hypertriglyceridemia* and need to bring your level down.

Causes of High Triglycerides

If you have a propensity to consume more calories than you use, then you are an expert at fat storage—and you have high triglycerides.

Far and away the most common causes of high triglycerides are obesity and a sedentary lifestyle.

Other common causes of high triglycerides include smoking, a very-high-carbohydrate diet, diabetes, chronic kidney failure, and excessive alcohol use. And, as with cholesterol, genetic factors play a role in triglyceride metabolism.

To sum it up, the most common causes of elevated triglycerides are

- Obesity and being overweight
- Physical inactivity
- Excessive alcohol intake
- A high-carbohydrate diet
- Smoking
- Certain medications (e.g., steroids, estrogen)
- Type 2 diabetes
- Chronic kidney failure
- Genetic factors

Triglycerides and Diabetes

Triglycerides, obesity, and diabetes are all very closely related. If you have increased abdominal fat (a figure shaped like an apple), you are at high risk for high triglycerides as well as insulin resistance, or Type 2 diabetes. That's because the fat cells in the abdomen release fatty acids into the blood more easily than fat in other parts of the body. The increased release of fatty acids leads to higher triglyceride levels and insulin resistance.

If you have high triglycerides, be on the lookout for low HDL cholesterol levels as well an insulin resistance and Type 2 diabetes.

Lowering Your Triglyceride Levels

Triglycerides are extremely responsive to healthy dietary and lifestyle changes. You can take a huge bite out of your elevated triglycerides level if you follow the Heart Smart formula.

When it comes to high triglycerides, you are in control. I have seen dramatic 200- to 300-point declines in triglyceride levels in just months when patients have made dietary changes, increased their exercise, and lost weight—without the use of drugs. It's worth your effort to lower your triglyceride levels to normal. It will lower your risk for heart attacks and cardiac death.

Eight Great Ways to Lower Your Triglyceride Levels

1. Lose weight.
2. Exercise often.
3. Reduce carbohydrates and sweets.
4. Reduce intake of bad fats/increase good fats.
5. Control your diabetes.
6. Eliminate alcohol.
7. Stop smoking.
8. Use triglyceride-lowering drugs (e.g., fibrates, statins, niacin).

I hope this triglyceride-lowering formula looks a bit familiar to you, it's very similar to the Heart Smart plans designed to help you lower your LDL cholesterol and raise your HDL cholesterol levels.

Focus on Dietary Changes

Since much of this ground has been covered in the last two sections and in Step Five, I am going to concentrate on the dietary aspects of lowering triglycerides. Triglycerides may be *the most responsive* component of your lipids to the effects of dietary changes, weight loss, and exercise. You can dramatically lower and even normalize your triglyceride levels in many cases with aggressive eating and lifestyle changes.

If your triglycerides are high, you've been making too many calorie deposits in your energy-storage bank. Now it's time to start making some withdrawals and put a lot of that stored energy to good use.

The first thing you should do toward your goal of lowering triglycerides is to reevaluate your diet. Check it to see if you're making any of the four major dietary mistakes that contribute to high triglycerides: eating too many carbohydrates, eating too many simple sugars, eating too much of the wrong kind of fat, and just eating too much.

Unless you exercise regularly, the average American diet (high-carbohydrate and high-calorie) gives you more fuel than you need. This will force your body to store the excess as fat, leading to high triglyceride levels. A high-fat diet raises your triglycerides, because fat is made of triglycerides. A high-sugar diet also will cause trouble—in fact, from a dietary standpoint, sugar has one of the greatest influences on triglyceride levels. Cutting out foods high in simple sugars has a major impact on lowering triglyceride levels.

The other major contributor to high triglyceride levels is alcohol, one of the most potent substances that can raise triglyceride levels. Alcohol raises triglyceride levels by both inhibiting the enzyme that breaks it down and by causing the liver to make more of it.

While mild to moderate alcohol intake may be associated with some heart-healthy benefits, those benefits may be overshadowed by the detrimental effects alcohol has on triglycerides. Drinking almost any alcohol (even as little as two to four ounces) raises triglyceride levels.

Triglyceride-Raising Foods (and Beverages) to Avoid

Saturated fats: Fats that are solid at room temperature, including lard, butter, shortening, and animal fats

Trans fats: Hydrogenated fats found in vegetable shortening, fried foods, fast foods, pies, cookies, crackers, commercially baked snacks, and margarine

Starches: Concentrated starchy foods such as potatoes, rice, pasta, bagels, chips, rolls, and white bread

Sugars: Jellies, candy, doughnuts, ice cream, all sugars, honey, jam, and jelly

Nonalcoholic drinks: Fruit juice, fruit punch, soda, sports drinks, sweetened coffee drinks

Alcohol: Beer, hard liquor, wine

Triglyceride-Smart Foods to Try

Protein: Lean meats, poultry without the skin, dried beans, egg whites, lentils, peas, soy products, and fish (e.g., salmon, mackerel, tuna)

Dairy: Low-fat yogurt, low-fat cheese, 1 percent or fat-free milk

Fat: One tablespoon canola, olive, or peanut oil a day, one-quarter cup nuts (e.g., peanuts, almonds, walnuts) five to seven days a week, olives, nut butter, avocados

Vegetables and fruits: Fresh only, no juices

Breads and cereals: Whole-grain breads and cereals, high-fiber cereal, unsweetened oatmeal, whole-grain crackers

---

Use Triglyceride-Lowering Drugs (e.g., Fibrates, Statins, Niacin)

When lifestyle and dietary changes aren't enough to lower your triglycerides to the target level, it's time to add one of the useful and proven medications available.

All three of the major classes of cholesterol-lowering drugs (see chapter 14) have some effect on lowering triglycerides. Since high triglycerides usually go hand in hand with other cholesterol problems, the best choice for you depends on your levels of LDL and HDL cholesterol and your overall risk of coronary heart disease.

Triglyceride-lowering drugs not only effectively lower your triglyceride levels, they also can save your life. One large clinical trial (called the VA-HIT Trial) studied patients with known heart disease who had mildly elevated triglyceride levels. Treatment with a class of medications known as fibrates lowered triglyceride levels by more than 30 percent (it had no effect on LDL cholesterol and only a very mild effect on HDL cholesterol), causing a dramatic 22 percent reduction in the participants' risk of dying from heart disease over a five-year period.

Fibrates

If high triglycerides are your primary lipid problem, then the first-line treatment choice is a group of medicines called fibric acids, or fibrates. Fibrates also are the first drug of choice if you have diabetes or the metabolic syndrome as well as high triglycerides and low HDL cholesterol. Fibrates can lower triglycerides by 25 to 50 percent and have been proven to lower your risk of heart attack and death from heart disease. Fibrates are part of a newly classified group of medicines called P-PARs (peroxisome proliferator activated receptors).

The fibrates work by increasing the level of lipoprotein lipase in your body, which helps break down the triglycerides and lower their blood level. Fibrates also raise good HDL cholesterol, decrease clotting activity, decrease artery and plaque inflammation, and improve insulin sensitivity. All of these benefits help fibrates lower triglyceride levels, reduce your chance of a heart attack, and save lives.

Statins

All cholesterol treatment guidelines make bad LDL cholesterol the first and most important factor to treat when it comes to preventing heart disease. If your LDL cholesterol and triglycerides are both elevated, then a statin drug should be used first. Statins have a very strong effect on bringing down LDL cholesterol as well as a smaller, but still beneficial, effect on bringing down triglyceride levels.

If your triglyceride levels are still elevated after you've reached your LDL cholesterol goal, then a second drug, such as a fibrate, can be added to the statin. Combination treatment with statins and fibrates can be very powerful and effective, though it increases the risk of liver and muscle side effects. If you begin a combination treatment, be sure to have your doctor monitor you very closely.

Niacin

Niacin is a fairly effective medication to use for lowering triglyceride levels. Niacin is a great choice for diabetics who have low HDL cholesterol along with elevated triglyceride levels. Niacin is commonly used in combination with a fibrate or statin drug to control triglyceride levels.

Summing It Up

LDL cholesterol is your prime target and number-one enemy when it comes to predicting, preventing, and treating coronary heart disease. LDL cholesterol is the "bad" cholesterol, and the optimal level is less than 100 mg/dL.

HDL cholesterol is the good cholesterol, and should be at least greater than 40 mg/dL, but the higher the better. Low levels of HDL cholesterol are a major independent risk factor for developing heart attacks and for dying from coronary heart disease.

Triglycerides are a measure of the fat proteins in the body, and elevated levels are an independent risk factor for heart disease. Normal triglyceride levels are less than 150 mg/dL. High triglyceride levels are caused by obesity, physical inactivity, excessive alcohol use, and high-fat and high-sugar diets.

Remember, close to 90 percent of cholesterol problems are due to completely controllable and preventable risk factors.

STEP THREE

Go High-Tech to Detect Heart Disease and Lower Your Risk

I t's the dawn of a new era in our fight against coronary heart disease: at long last, emerging cardiovascular technology is focusing on detecting heart disease in its *earliest* stages—even *before* symptoms develop. This paradigm shift is changing the way we prevent and treat heart disease from one in which we're *reactive* to one in which we're *proactive*.

Step Three of the Heart Smart detection and prevention program introduces you to the hottest cardiovascular technology and the latest science that are driving this paradigm shift. From understanding new cardiac risk factors to utilizing new lab tests and multimillion-dollar high-tech imaging studies, you'll learn about the latest and greatest tools—and how to use them—to help you determine your cardiac risk and prevent heart attacks.

In this section, you'll get an up-to-date look at the new markers that can help you predict your cardiac risk. You'll find out why routine cholesterol tests can be so misleading and how to avoid being the next "completely healthy" victim of a stealthy heart attack. From C-reactive protein to homocysteine, we'll look at special cholesterol factors, clotting, infection, and inflammatory factors that increase your heart attack risk.

Additionally, I'll uncover, perhaps for the first time, the truth about stress testing. While stress tests are a valuable weapon, there are potential downsides of this procedure as well as one particularly dirty little secret.

Finally, we'll look at the latest in imaging and stress tests, which look both within your heart and beyond to detect early coronary heart disease.

I will also tell you all about the future of cardiac testing and the ultimate, one-stop heart test.

Chapter 7

Digging Deeper into Your Risk

Inflammation, Infection, and Beyond: Which
Emerging Factors Should You Be Tested For?

Peter had a heart attack when he was just forty-four years old. He didn't have high blood pressure, he didn't have diabetes, he didn't smoke, and his total, LDL, and HDL cholesterol levels were normal. In fact, before his heart attack, Peter didn't seem to have any cardiac risk factors at all. By all accounts he was the picture of good health.

Why Did Peter Have a Heart Attack?

When I saw Peter following his heart attack, I told him that though his heart attack seemed a mystery, heart attacks don't occur without a reason. I was sure that if we looked in the right places we would uncover the cause of his heart attack. Peter was surprised to learn that up to 10 to 15 percent of heart attack victims don't have any of the traditional cardiac risk factors, and almost half have a normal or near-normal LDL cholesterol level.

Because Peter was in that 15 percent, we turned our attention to a new group of cardiac risk factors called "emerging" heart disease risk factors. These factors can occur alone or in combination with traditional cardiac risk factors, but either way they can significantly increase your risk for coronary heart disease and heart attacks. Emerging risks include *cholesterol*, *clotting*, *infectious*, and *inflammatory* factors.

Screening for many of these emerging risk factors becomes a critical step in determining your cardiac risk and in developing an effective treatment plan for coronary heart disease. In my opinion these tests are too often misunderstood and underutilized. If you're interested in knowing the complete story of your cardiac risk, you need to learn about these important emerging factors and get yourself tested for all that may affect you (later, I'll tell you how you and your doctor can decide which tests to have).

Some of the tests in this chapter are specialized blood tests that may not be available at your local commercial labs. They may or may not be completely covered by your insurance, depending on your diagnosis. I strongly recommend that you work with your doctor, insurance company, and lab prior to having the tests.

Now let's look at each emerging factor.

Emerging Cardiac Risk Factors

Cholesterol Factors

- *HDL2b:* For a more in-depth look at how good your good cholesterol really is.

- *Lipoprotein* (a)*:* A dangerous and often overlooked cause of heart attacks.

- LDL *particle size* or LDL *pattern:* Not all "bad" cholesterol is created equal: Size matters, and the test for this factor tells you what your LDL particle size is.

- *Apolipoprotein B:* Gives you a more accurate measurement of your bad cholesterol.

Clotting Factors

- *Fibrinogen:* A clotting factor that may increase your heart attack risk.

Inflammatory, Infectious, and Other Factors

- *C-reactive protein:* A sensitive marker of coronary inflammation and a great predictor of future heart attacks.

- *Lp-PLA$_2$:* An arterial inflammation factor that predicts your cardiac risk.

- *Homocysteine:* A controversial marker of heart risk.

- *Chlamydia pneumoniae:* A type of "bug" that may put your arteries at risk for cholesterol attack.

Emerging Cholesterol Factors

As I discussed in chapter 4, the fasting cholesterol panel is an excellent cardiac-risk screening tool that I recommend for everyone over age twenty. The panel provides you with your total cholesterol, HDL cholesterol, LDL cholesterol, and triglyceride levels.

However, though the screening cholesterol panel is a great start, we can do much better. Recent advances in laboratory technology keep pushing the envelope, making cholesterol testing more sophisticated, more thorough, and more accurate than ever before. Here are few of the more important subcomponents of cholesterol to be aware of.

HDL: 2b or Not 2b? That Is the Question.

From reading chapter 6 you know that HDL is the "good" cholesterol. High levels of HDL cholesterol protect your heart and keep you at low risk for heart attacks. So how can some people with normal HDL cholesterol levels, like Peter above, still have heart attacks?

The reason is that not all HDL cholesterol components protect your heart equally: some are more protective than others, making a normal HDL reading occasionally misleading. So, unfortunately, even if you have all the HDL in the world, if it's the wrong kind of HDL it's not going to help protect your heart.

Currently, we know of five major subclasses of HDL that roam around in your body: HDL2a, HDL2b, HDL3a, HDL3b, and HDL3c. The subtype HDL2b is the most important and most protective HDL cholesterol for your heart. The higher your HDL2b level, the lower your cardiac risk; conversely, the lower your HDL2b level, the higher your risk.

HDL2b cholesterol protects your heart in two ways: by releasing antioxidants to protect your endothelium (the inner lining of your heart arteries) and by driving *the reverse cholesterol transport system*. As you read in chapter 6, HDL takes bad cholesterol out of your arteries and delivers it back to the liver for disposal. The reverse cholesterol transport system drives this protective function.

Should You Have Your HDL2b Checked?

Not everyone needs to be tested for HDL2b levels. If you already have very low HDL levels or if you have a high HDL level and no other cardiac risk factors, you don't need to worry about checking your HDL2b level. There are many situations, however, where checking the "quality" of your HDL levels with a HDL2b level can play an important role.

I recommend checking your level in the following situations:

- If you have a borderline HDL level and are trying to decide on whether to take medications to treat your HDL.
- If you developed coronary artery disease younger than age fifty.
- If you have a family history of premature coronary artery disease.
- If you developed coronary artery disease with a "normal" or high HDL level and have no other cardiac risk factors.

If you fit into one of these categories, be sure that your HDL cholesterol is protecting you the way you think it is.

If you decide to take the test and learn that you have a high level of HDL2b (greater than 20 percent of total HDL in men and greater than 35 percent of HDL in women), you can rest assured that your reverse cholesterol transport system is fully operational. If the level is high you probably do not need to recheck it in the future unless there is a drastic change in your lifestyle. A low HDL2b level should be tracked with serial measurements until it normalizes.

Raising Your HDL2b Level: It's in Your Hands

How can you raise your HDL2b level if it's low and not providing the protection you need? Diet and lifestyle changes will go a long way in solving the problem and help you to maintain a high level once it's reached. The most important things you can do are maintain an ideal weight, increase the time you spend exercising, and limit carbohydrate and simple sugar intake.

For more information on raising HDL levels see chapter 6.

Lipoprotein (a): The Hidden Killer

Looking for, finding, and treating elevated lipoprotein (a), also known as Lp(a) (pronounced "lp little a"), has changed my practice and changed the lives of many of my patients. Lp(a) is a hidden killer, and it is not part of the routine lipid panel. Its level is detected only if your doctor specifically looks for it.

Chris, a friend of mine, is a candidate for having his Lp(a) checked:

While taking a ski break on top of a mountain in Utah this year, my old friend Chris asked me why doctors couldn't figure out what causes heart attacks. I told him we pretty much know what causes heart attacks, and went through all the cardiac risk factors. Chris had his reservations: he pessimistically said that his uncle had been perfectly healthy, hadn't had any cardiac risk factors, and still had died suddenly at age fifty-one from a heart attack. Chris wanted to know if he could be next.

I asked Chris what his uncle's Lp(a) level had been. Chris had never heard about emerging cardiac risk factors, and definitely not about Lp(a). I told him that "healthy" people who had had a heart attack simply had not dug deep enough to uncover all their risks. I then told Chris all about Lp(a) and suggested that he get it checked.

Almost a third of people who suffer a *premature* heart attack (before age fifty-five in men or sixty-five in women) have an elevated Lp(a) level—and they don't know their level is high. A high Lp(a) level increases your risk of coronary heart disease by an incredible 200 to 300 percent *even if your good and bad cholesterol levels are normal.* High Lp(a) is an extremely dangerous cardiac risk factor that requires specialized treatment.

What Is Lp(a)?

Lp(a) is similar to bad LDL cholesterol except it's even more dangerous! That's because it has an additional clot-producing protein attached to it. Lp(a) consists of a particle of LDL cholesterol linked to apolipoprotein(a), which has a similar structure to plasminogen, which plays a central role in clotting and clot formation inside your arteries.

Lp(a), therefore, is a double threat to your heart because it promotes cardiovascular disease and heart attacks in two ways: its LDL cholesterol particle promotes cholesterol plaque formation (atherogenesis), and its apolipoprotein(a) particle promotes clotting (thrombogenesis).

Normal Lp(a) Levels

Lp(a) is unique because it's the one cardiac risk factor that you don't have much control over. Elevated Lp(a) levels appear to be driven more by genetics—you can thank your parents if your Lp(a) is elevated—than by lifestyle factors. Unfortunately, diet and exercise have little effect on your Lp(a), and it's resistant to most cholesterol-lowering drugs.

What is a normal level? Most doctors and labs consider less than 30 mg/dL of Lp(a) to be in the normal range.

Treating Lp(a)

Detecting an elevated Lp(a) level is easy enough if your doctor actually looks for it; treating a high level can be a little more challenging. The lifestyle factors such as diet, weight loss, and exercise that play such a central role in treating traditional cardiac risk factors have little impact on lowering Lp(a) levels.

To lower your Lp(a) level you have to turn to drug therapy; the "go to" drug for doing so is niacin. But you need to take more than a little niacin; you need a high dose—usually 2 to 4 g/day.

High-dose niacin can effectively lower Lp(a) levels by up to 50 percent. Unfortunately, the drug's side effects (mainly the niacin "flush," a hot, burning sensation of the skin) significantly limit the number of people who can tolerate the higher amount. Of all the patients I have treated with niacin to lower their Lp(a), only about a third have been able to tolerate the side effects of the high dose. The dose of niacin that's best for you lowers your Lp(a) level; you may be able to get away with using lower doses.

If you discover that you have an elevated Lp(a) level and you can't handle a high dose of niacin, your best bet is to live a heart-healthy lifestyle so that you minimize all your other cardiac risk factors for coronary heart disease.

Should You Have Your Lp(a) Checked?

As I told my friend Chris, "healthy" people who have heart attacks just didn't look deeply enough to find their cardiac risk factors. If they had, many would have found that they had an elevated Lp(a) level.

Many "experts," however, do not recommend that everyone check his or her Lp(a) level. They argue that for people at the lowest end of the cardiac risk spectrum (no family history of heart disease, normal weight, normal good and bad cholesterol levels, normal blood pressure, normal blood sugar levels, not a smoker), checking their Lp(a) level probably does not add much to their cardiac risk evaluation.

Others don't check it because even if your level is elevated, the treatment options are somewhat limited. My approach to checking Lp(a) levels is more aggressive than most national guidelines and experts recommend. I believe that since Lp(a) is primarily determined by genetics, there is no way to know if yours is elevated unless you check for it. I recommend that all my patients have at least one screening test to check their Lp(a) level. If it's high, then I treat it and track it. If it's normal, then I typically don't recheck it.

Despite the differences, most doctors agree that certain groups of patients should have their Lp(a) checked. If you developed coronary heart disease at an early age or if you have a strong family history of premature coronary heart disease, you should be tested to see if your Lp(a) level is high.

Heart Smart Lp(a) Alert

If you or one of your relatives developed coronary artery disease before age fifty, or if you developed coronary artery disease without having any (or many) of the traditional cardiac risk factors, you should ask your doctor to have your Lp(a) level tested right away; special lab testing is required.

Lp(a) and C-reactive protein, in my estimation, are the two most important emergent cardiac risk markers to determine.

LDL Particle Size or LDL Pattern: Size Really Matters

Since LDL cholesterol size is not part of the routine cholesterol panel, most people don't ever think or worry about LDL size as a factor when it comes to coronary heart disease. It turns out, though, that this risk factor's size plays a major role in your risk for a heart attack. The smaller the particle size, the greater the threat LDL cholesterol is to your heart. That's because the smaller particles can burrow their way into your heart arteries more easily than big LDL particles.

The most dangerous type of LDL cholesterol is known as *small, dense LDL cholesterol*. This type of LDL cholesterol increases your risk for coronary heart disease by up to six times. Small LDL cholesterol is an independent risk factor for coronary heart disease, even if your total LDL cholesterol is normal.

What Causes LDL to Be Small and Dangerous?

Many of the common diet and lifestyle factors that contribute to many of the cardiac risk factors also cause your LDL cholesterol to be small. Obesity, smoking, a sedentary lifestyle, and diabetes have all been associated with small LDL cholesterol size. Genetics also play an important role; many people with small, dense LDL cholesterol have no other cardiac risk factors, and have only their parents to thank for this dangerous condition that causes heart attacks.

It's the Pattern That Really Matters

To find out the size of your LDL cholesterol particles, specialized cholesterol testing is needed. But rather than report particle size, most labs report your LDL cholesterol pattern.

If most of your LDL type is "small and dense," you have *LDL pattern B* (the dangerous type). LDL pattern B is not only a marker for coronary heart disease; it is also a marker of more progressive and unstable coronary heart disease. If most of your LDL particles are "large," then you have the less dangerous *LDL pattern A*.

Reversing LDL Pattern B

Unlike Lp(a), LDL pattern B is very responsive to lifestyle changes; it not only can be reversed but can even be changed to the safer LDL pattern A. Losing weight, increasing the time you spend exercising, and following a low-fat, low-carbohydrate diet can increase the size of your LDL cholesterol. Several medications also can help make this change, including nicotinic acid and the cholesterol medications known as fibrates.

Should You Have Your LDL Size and Pattern Checked?

As with many of the other emerging risk factors, I tend to be more aggressive in checking LDL size than most national guidelines recommend. I believe that everyone with borderline to elevated LDL cholesterol levels, everyone who has developed coronary artery disease at a young age, and everyone who has developed coronary artery disease without any (or just a few) of the traditional cardiac risk factors should be tested for LDL cholesterol size and pattern.

In my opinion, you never can have too much information about your cholesterol and the other risk factors that contribute to heart attacks.

Apolipoprotein B: A More Direct Measurement of Bad Cholesterol

Measuring LDL cholesterol is not as accurate as we would like it to be. In fact, the routine cholesterol panel doesn't even directly measure LDL cholesterol.

Several factors limit our ability to measure LDL cholesterol levels, the biggest being that LDL cholesterol is an *indirect* rather than a *direct* measurement. Indirectly measuring LDL leads to inaccurate measurement, and sometime measurements can't even be obtained; this can happen if you have very high triglyceride levels, diabetes, or liver or kidney disease. Techniques are available to directly measure LDL cholesterol levels, but they are not used regularly because they are expensive and there are no universal standards.

Another major limitation on measuring total LDL cholesterol is that while we are able to measure your total LDL cholesterol, the measurement doesn't tell *how many* LDL particles you have. You may have a small number of large LDL particles (LDL pattern A) or a large number of smaller LDL particles (LDL pattern B), but whichever it is, you still have the same total amount of LDL cholesterol.

If you really want a complete measurement of all your LDL cholesterol, you need to measure your apolipoprotein B, or apo B, level.

The Pizza Comparison

How does the apo B measurement work? Think of total LDL cholesterol levels in terms of a pizza. The entire pizza represents your total LDL cholesterol level. Whether you cut it in half and have two large pieces of pizza or slice it up into thirty smaller pieces, you have the same amount of pizza. Your total LDL cholesterol, just like that pizza, is the same no matter how you slice it.

The most important thing for you to know, however, is how many LDL particles are in that total cholesterol, and that's what the apo B test allows you to measure. As we talked about above, a large number of small particles—think of it as a pizza cut into a lot of small slices—is much more dangerous than a smaller number of big pieces—like a pizza cut into just a few slices. The small particles can move more easily into your heart arteries.

What Is Apo B?

Apo B is protein that sits on top of LDL cholesterol particles; each LDL particle the liver produces has one apo B protein attached to it. Because of the link, measuring how much apo B you have provides a direct and accurate way to gauge the number of LDL particles you have. Apo B is associated with dangerous oxidation and inflammation that occurs when LDL cholesterol attacks your arteries.

Normal apo B levels are less than 80 mg/dL, although some experts recommend that they should be less than 60 mg/dL. Elevated apo B levels are associated with an increased risk of fatal heart attacks and are a proven independent risk factor for coronary heart disease.

Should You Have Your Apo B Level Checked?

Apo B levels have a unique niche in determining your cardiac risk. I recommend that you have your apo B level checked if you have inaccurate or immeasurable LDL cholesterol levels. This happens commonly in the face of very high triglyceride levels or if you have kidney or liver disease.

Apo B levels may also be useful if you are at moderate to high risk for coronary heart disease, have premature coronary heart disease, or have a family history of premature heart disease.

Emerging Clotting Factors

A major part of the process of atherosclerosis and heart attacks is related to blood clotting. In fact, a massive blood clotting reaction is the final straw that causes a heart attack.

Internal blood clotting is a normal and useful process. Blood clotting factors circulate in your blood looking for injuries in your arteries and clot the blood to prevent bleeding. This is good news if you cut your finger but bad news when blood is clotted inside one of your heart arteries at the site of injury caused by a cholesterol plaque. Clotting inside your heart arteries is a life-threatening event.

There are many different types of clotting factors circulating in the blood; however, only fibrinogen will be covered here because it is one of the most studied clotting factors and is readily detected by a blood test.

Fibrinogen

Fibrinogen is a protein that is produced by the liver and travels in the bloodstream. Fibrinogen is essential for the clotting of blood. Blood clots form when fibrinogen is broken down into fibrin by an enzyme called thrombin. Fibrin then forms a complex lattice that platelets stick to, causing clot formation.

Fibrinogen, as well as other clotting factors, is definitely involved in heart disease; in fact, the combination of elevated fibrinogen levels and elevated LDL cholesterol levels may increase the risk of cardiovascular disease sixfold.

Should You Have Your Fibrinogen Level Checked?

High levels of circulating fibrinogen are strongly associated with cardiovascular disease, but research has not yet been able to clarify if this association has a bearing on your overall risk. One day the fibrinogen level may become a routine part of heart disease screening, but at this point I do not recommend routine screening of your fibrinogen. Currently there is no direct treatment for elevated fibrinogen levels and, at least in my experience, knowing the level doesn't add much to your cardiovascular risk evaluation.

Emerging Inflammatory, Infectious, and Other Factors

One of the biggest discoveries in heart disease over the past decade is that atherosclerosis is primarily an inflammatory process gone out of control. This inflammatory process inside the heart arteries can now be quantified with incredible new blood tests that are here to stay. In addition, infectious and other new measurable factors also may play a significant role in determining cardiac risk. This section reviews some of the hottest topics in heart disease prevention and cardiology today.

C-Reactive Protein: A Powerful Predictor of Risk!

C-reactive protein (CRP) is a hot topic in cardiology and heart disease prevention research. It is an *acute phase reactant* that is produced by the liver in response to any inflammation, which can be caused by infection, injury, or stress. CRP levels are commonly elevated in patients with rheumatoid arthritis, periodontal disease, and many other causes of inflammation. It has come to be used as a marker of heart disease because researchers have now positively identified atherosclerosis as an inflammatory process; arterial inflammation equals arterial damage.

Testing for CRP

The best test when looking for elevated CRP is a blood test known as a high-sensitivity CRP (hs-CRP). It can be performed at the same time as a cholesterol panel, but it is not part of the routine cholesterol panel. If the result shows that your hs-CRP level is less than 1 mg/L, you have minimal or no inflammation in your heart arteries and are at low risk for having a heart attack. If it is above 3 mg/L, you are at a much higher risk of a cardiac event—you're five times more likely to have a heart attack than if you had a low CRP level. A level between puts you at a moderately increased risk.

Since CRP levels can be elevated in many conditions, make sure there are no other inflammatory processes if you decide to take the test (see box). Most experts recommend taking at least two CRP tests a few weeks apart to help make sure the result is accurate and not influenced by another underlying condition.

Should You Have Your CRP Level Checked?

Elevated levels of high-sensitivity C-reactive protein are associated with higher risks of heart attack, stroke, peripheral vascular disease, and sudden death. Knowing your level will provide important information about your cardiac risk to supplement what you learn from your cholesterol measurement alone. A growing number of experts now strongly argue for the routine use of CRP screening to identify if you are at risk for heart disease. By testing for CRP you may be able to detect the inflammatory atherosclerotic process *before* it causes symptoms and does a lot of damage.

Using CRP Levels to Predict Future Heart Events

Most studies show that elevated CRP levels are much more effective at predicting heart attacks and cardiac death than elevated LDL cholesterol levels, for healthy people as well as for those who already have coronary heart disease. A few of the most recent clinical trials showed that:

- CRP >2.0 mg/L is twice as effective a predictor of future coronary artery disease risk as elevated LDL cholesterol.

- Female patients with elevated CRP levels and *low* LDL levels were the highest risk group for future heart events. The risk to this group would have been completely missed if only traditional cholesterol levels had been checked.

- The higher the CRP level, the more likely a plaque will become unstable and rupture.

- Elevated CRP levels increase your relative risk of a future heart attack by more than three times; when combined with abnormal cholesterol levels the risk is raised to more than *five times*.

Clinical Evidence Supporting C-Reactive Protein Testing

Two important trials—the REVERSAL (Reversal of Atherosclerosis with Aggressive Lipid Lowering) Trial and the PROVE IT:TIMI 22 (Pravastatin or Atorvastatin Evaluation and Infection Therapy—Thrombolysis in Myocardial Infarction 22) Trial—both show strong evidence that lowering CRP levels with the statin drugs is associated with improved outcomes and lower clinical cardiac event rates *regardless* of LDL cholesterol levels. When discussing these trials, Peter Libby, M.D., chief of cardiovascular medicine at Brigham and Women's Hospital in Boston, said, "That C-reactive protein can be a prospective gauge of risk I think is settled beyond a doubt."

With all that said, there still are some limitations in using the CRP test. If you have absolutely no cardiac risk factors and are at low risk for coronary heart disease, the CRP level will not add very much to your risk evaluation.

If, on the other hand, you are at moderate or high risk for coronary heart disease based on traditional risk factors, the CRP level can add important insight to your risk. CRP levels should be taken into consideration with all other cardiac risk factors. It can be a very helpful test when used appropriately.

The bottom line is that there is still some debate about who should be tested for CRP level, how often they should be tested, and whether treatment should be directed specifically toward lowering CRP. Most experts agree, however, that arterial inflammation plays a central role in atherosclerosis and heart attacks, so I urge my patients to err on the side of caution. Knowing and tracking your CRP level is safe and relatively inexpensive. Any extra information you have about your cardiac risk will only help you in the long term.

Treating High CRP Levels

As noted above, we now have proof that lowering CRP levels is associated with improved cardiac outcomes. Controlling your diet, exercising, and losing weight are the best ways to lower your CRP level if it's high. If those don't work, the statin drugs have been shown to drive CRP levels down by as much as 25 percent.

If you currently are being treated for coronary heart disease, you may require serial measurements of your CRP level, just as you do of your cholesterol levels, to ensure that treatment is bringing your CRP down to normal.

CRP-Lowering and Statin Drugs

Groundbreaking new data show that you can *dramatically lower* your risk of a heart attack by lowering your CRP level with the statin drugs.

Lipoprotein-associated Phospholipase A$_2$: The PLAC Test

Looking for evidence of ongoing inflammation is going to play a major role in the detection and treatment of heart disease from now on. In addition to using the CRP test to look for inflammation in the arteries, you can use another brand-new way to evaluate your cardiac risk: measuring an enzyme in the blood called lipoprotein-associated phospholipase A$_2$, also known as Lp-PLA$_2$.

Lp-PLA$_2$ is an enzyme produced by specialized white blood cells called macrophages. The enzyme, which is a marker of vascular inflammation, flocks to areas of vascular damage where atherosclerosis is taking place. Lp-PLA$_2$ activity is increased and levels rise as oxidized LDL cholesterol begins attacking your artery walls. Lp-PLA$_2$ also helps attract other inflammatory mediators to the area of attack.

Two recent major trials evaluating cholesterol and cardiac risk—the West of Scotland Prevention Study and the Atherosclerosis in Risk Communities Trials—identified Lp-PLA$_2$ as a potent predictor of cardiac risk. The greatest increase in cardiac risk was seen in patients with the highest Lp-PLA$_2$ levels and LDL cholesterol less than 130 mg/dL. This group of patients had two to three times the risk of having coronary heart disease than patients with lower Lp-PLA$_2$ levels.

Should You Have Your Lp-PLA$_2$ Level Checked?

Like CRP, Lp-PLA$_2$ is a marker of coronary inflammation. Your level can be checked with a test known as the PLAC test. If your level is high, it is possible to lower it with fibrates and statin drugs, but it is not yet clear, as it is with lowering CRP levels, that lowering your Lp-PLA$_2$ lowers your

risk of a heart attack. Proponents of the PLAC test think that it will ultimately replace the CRP test because the CRP test is a marker of nonspe-
cific inflammation, whereas the Lp-PLA$_2$ test is a more direct marker of
arterial inflammation only. At this point, until new clinical data with the
PLAC test show clear evidence of improved risk information and
improved outcomes by lowering Lp-PLA$_2$ levels, I recommend sticking
with the CRP test.

Homocysteine: Marker or Risk Factor for Heart Disease?

There is a definite association between elevated homocysteine levels
(hyperhomocysteinemia) and coronary heart disease, stroke, deep venous
thrombosis, and vascular disease. There is large debate, however, as to
whether high homocysteine levels cause coronary heart disease or just act
as a *marker* for coronary heart disease. It's the classic chicken-and-egg
question: which came first?

What Is Homocysteine?

Homocysteine is an amino acid that is involved in making many life-sus-
taining proteins for your body. Homocysteine levels are easily measured
in a blood sample by most laboratories, though it is not part of the routine cholesterol panel and needs to be specially ordered. High-protein
meals can significantly affect homocysteine levels, so you need to fast for
ten to twelve hours before the test. A normal homocysteine level for most
labs is <10 micromoles per liter.

Chronic kidney failure, hypothyroidism, and pernicious anemia are
all associated with high homocysteine levels. These levels also can be elevated with increasing age, menopause, smoking, prolonged alcohol abuse,
and with use of some drugs, such as niacin. However, homocysteine levels are usually kept in check because the amino acid is broken down into
safer subcomponents by the vitamin cofactors folic acid, vitamin B$_{12}$
(cobalamin), and vitamin B$_6$ (pyridoxine).

While these vitamins are available in pill form, there are a number of
natural food sources that can supply you with all the breakdown power
they provide. For example, folate (folic acid) is found in dried beans,
lentils, peas, whole wheat, broccoli, spinach, and beets. Animal products
such as eggs, cheese, and milk products supply vitamin B$_{12}$, and vitamin B$_6$
can be found in both animal and plant sources.

Does Elevated Homocysteine Cause Heart Disease?

While clinical studies dating back to the 1960s have shown that elevated homocysteine levels are associated with coronary artery disease, there is only marginal proof that homocysteine is a true predictor of heart attacks. To date there is no convincing or overwhelming proof that lowering homocysteine with medication saves lives.

Some studies suggest that elevated homocysteine levels are as important at predicting heart disease as elevated cholesterol levels are. Others show no real predictive value. A recent review published in the *Journal of the American Medical Association*, which looked back at thirty years of clinical testing of homocysteine, showed at most a modest independent predictive value connecting elevated homocysteine levels with coronary heart disease and stroke in healthy individuals.

Of great concern, however, are a few studies that show on average that people with heart disease and high levels of homocysteine are at a two to three times higher risk of having a heart attack and heart procedures than people who have lower homocysteine levels.

High homocysteine levels, however, may contribute to atherosclerosis by a number of different mechanisms: endothelial dysfunction, artery vasospasm, and the promotion of platelet stickiness and clot formation.

Treating Elevated Homocysteine

If you have or if you are at high risk of coronary heart disease and have elevated homocysteine levels, you need to consider treatment. Lowering elevated homocysteine levels is safe and effective with the vitamin cofactors folic acid, vitamin B_{12}, and vitamin B_6. With this combination treatment, levels may drop by as much as 70 percent.

If you require medication therapy, a starting dose of supplements is folate, 2.5 mgs; vitamin B_{12}, 1 mg; and vitamin B_6, 25 mgs. Treatment is indefinite, and follow-up tests for homocysteine levels will be needed to determine how effective treatment has been.

Should You Have Your Homocysteine Level Checked?

The latest recommendation from the experts who wrote the ATP III guidelines is *not* to routinely check the homocysteine level as part of the risk assessment for heart disease.

I believe, however, that checking and aggressively treating elevated homocysteine levels play a very important role if you fit into one of two groups:

1. You were diagnosed with heart disease at an early age (prior to age fifty) or you have a family history of premature heart disease.

2. You have coronary heart disease but none of the traditional risk factors for it.

If you're in one of those categories, I recommend erring on the side of caution by checking and, if found, treating elevated homocysteine until more definitive, ongoing trials point us in one direction or another.

Chlamydia Pneumoniae: Do Antibiotics Play a Role in Fighting Heart Disease?

Could the cold you had last winter have triggered your heart attack?

Some data suggest that it might have. A link has been established between certain infectious agents and coronary heart disease. *Chlamydia pneumoniae*, *Helicobacter pylori*, CMV, and the herpes simplex virus are all being evaluated as possible infectious triggers for the development of coronary heart disease. And while it's not yet clear how infectious agents cause coronary artery disease, the prevailing thought is that they promote endothelial dysfunction and local inflammation that contribute to the initiation of atherosclerosis.

By far and away the agent that has been studied most as a potential cause of atherosclerosis is *Chlamydia pneumoniae*. Researchers have linked *Chlamydia* infections to both acute myocardial infarctions as well as chronic coronary artery disease. In addition, promising animal research has shown evidence of *Chlamydia* infection directly in the atherosclerotic plaque in forty-four out of forty-seven cases. However, the research is far from conclusive at this stage, and there are just as many studies that do not show an infectious link to coronary heart disease as those that do show a link.

Should You Be Tested for *Chlamydia Pneumoniae*?

Antibody testing to detect evidence of Chlamydia infections is relatively cheap and widely available. At this point in time, however, I do not recommend routine testing for *Chlamydia pneumoniae* or any other infectious agents during the evaluation or treatment of coronary artery disease.

Two excellent studies reported in the *New England Journal of Medicine* in 2005 concluded that treating people who have coronary artery disease with antibiotics to suppress *Chlamydia pneumoniae* is *not effective and does not change cardiovascular outcomes.* The infection–heart disease connection is still in its earliest stages, but thus far there is not convincing or consistent data to suggest that detecting or treating infectious agents will lower your cardiac risk.

Whatever Happened to Peter?

Remember Peter, who I told you about at the beginning of this chapter? He was confused about heart disease causes and wondered how he could have had a heart attack without seeming to have had any cardiac risk factors.

As it turned out, Peter did have some cardiac risk factors; he just hadn't dug deeply enough to find them before his heart attack. I told Peter that he should have some special blood tests done to look specifically for the emerging cardiac risk factors. We found that he had two major cholesterol problems that had caused his heart attack—but they had been completely missed by routine cholesterol screening.

While it was true that Peter's overall LDL cholesterol was not elevated, we discovered that he was loaded with the small, dense LDL cholesterol that can be so dangerous. Peter had tested positive for the LDL cholesterol pattern B.

In addition to that, Peter also had elevated levels of the heart attack–causing Lp(a). These two factors put Peter at high risk for heart disease, although he had believed he was in great heart health.

Since learning about his two risk factors, Peter has been on a heart-healthy diet, taking niacin and exercising regularly. The treatment has changed his LDL pattern from the dangerous B to the less dangerous A type, and his Lp(a) levels have normalized. Peter now champions early screening for the emerging cardiac risk factors.

Summing It Up

It is critical that you take advantage of every tool at your disposal to help you prevent heart attacks and fight coronary heart disease. That includes testing for the emerging cardiac risk factors. Whether occurring alone or in combination with traditional risk factors, the emerging cardiac risk factors may substantially increase your cardiac risk.

Don't fall victim to a stealthy heart attack or be one of those people whose friends end up saying, "But he was so healthy; I can't believe he had a heart attack and died so suddenly." Simple lab tests that detect the new factors can help to save your life.

Chapter 8

The Truth about Stress Tests

*What They Can and Can't Tell You
about Your Cardiac Risk*

Stress tests play a central role in the evaluation and treatment of chest pain and coronary artery disease. They do right now, and they'll continue to do so in the future.

Stress tests, however, should come with a warning label. If you're not careful they can give you a false sense of security and leave you at high risk for heart attacks and sudden cardiac death.

There are two important things you need to understand about the stress test: what it tells you and what it *doesn't* tell you. In this chapter I'm going to take you beyond the basics that you find in other books and give you the complete story—the only book in which you'll find it—about the limitations and potential *downsides* as well as the benefits of stress testing.

Scott, one of my patients, learned about the pitfalls of stress testing the hard way.

Scott was an active, healthy forty-seven-year-old with a family history of heart disease and high cholesterol. Scott asked his doctor if there were any tests he could take to help make sure his heart was doing okay.

Scott's primary care physician recommended a "screening" stress test as part of his routine physical examination. The results of the test were perfect—Scott was doing great, and it looked like he had nothing to worry about regarding his heart. The positive results gave Scott a great feeling of confidence that he was doing everything right and that his heart was in good condition.

Three weeks later, Scott's distraught wife called to tell me he had suffered a major heart attack at work. He had been rushed to the hospital unconscious, had emergency heart surgery, and was in critical condition in the coronary care unit.

His wife asked me if Scott had been telling the truth when he told her that his stress test had been great. I confirmed that Scott's test had indeed been normal just three weeks before.

What had happened? Was the stress test wrong? Could anything else have been done to prevent Scott's heart attack?

This chapter will tell you exactly how this tragedy happened, why it could easily happen to you, and how to avoid it.

What Is a Stress Test?

A stress test is a common diagnostic test performed by cardiologists to evaluate chest pain, assess your cardiac risk, and determine if you have any *major* blockages in your heart arteries (the test does not detect mild or moderate heart disease); it is safe, noninvasive, quick, and 60 to 90 percent accurate in detecting severe coronary heart disease.

During the test the patient exercises on a treadmill or is given medication to make his or her heart think it's exercising. The test increases the heart's need for oxygen in order to evaluate its response to the increased workload. During a stress test your heart is monitored for changes in blood flow both at rest and during exercise. A decrease in blood flow during stress signifies a major cholesterol blockage in at least one of the heart arteries.

The Nuts and Bolts of the Stress Test

Stress tests may be done in the hospital or in your doctor's office. A qualified nurse or technologist often performs the test, with a doctor nearby and available if needed. Throughout the test, EKG and blood pressure monitors constantly analyze your heart rate, rhythm, and blood pressure.

The exercise is done on a motorized treadmill in a series of three-minute periods of advancing speed and grade (known as the "Bruce Protocol"). The test is completed when you reach your target heart rate, develop chest pain, or can no longer keep exercising.

Why Should You Have a Stress Test?

Stress tests are used for a number of reasons, but the primary indications are to evaluate chest pain, evaluate the effectiveness of heart disease treatment, help determine a safe level of exercise, and evaluate your cardiac risk.

Chest Pain Evaluation

The most common reason to have a stress test is to evaluate chest pain symptoms. As you may recall from chapter 2, it can be challenging to figure out the underlying cause of chest pain.

Stress tests help determine whether chest pain is caused by coronary heart disease. A normal stress test result points toward other causes of chest pain (musculoskeletal or gastrointestinal), while an abnormal or "positive" result points toward blocked heart arteries as the cause of chest pain.

Stress tests also are used to evaluate any of the other symptoms commonly associated with coronary heart disease, including shortness of breath and palpitations.

Treatment Effectiveness

Stress tests are a good way to track the effectiveness of coronary artery disease treatment. Whether you have been treated with medications or with surgery (angioplasty, stents, or bypass surgery), serial stress tests are often used to learn how your heart is responding to treatment.

Exercise Level

Some people have significant coronary artery disease but don't know that they do. If they start an exercise routine after a long period of inactivity, it's possible for them to do serious damage to their heart.

Diabetics, women, the elderly, and any couch potato benefit from taking a stress test prior to starting an exercise program. The results of the test will help them determine an appropriate, safe workout level and make sure they have no hidden coronary heart disease.

Cardiac Risk

Stress tests are commonly used to assess a person's cardiac risk. Many physicians include stress tests as part of their routine screening for their forty- to fifty-year-old patients. However, while stress tests do give some hints as to cardiac fitness, they should not be used alone as a gauge of cardiac risk because they leave many people with a false sense of security about their heart health.

Types of Stress Tests

All stress tests have the same goal; it's how they reach it that differs.

Your heart can be "stressed" with exercise or with special medications that stimulate your heart to increase its oxygen demands. Exercise is the preferred method for the evaluation of coronary heart disease. It is ideal because it is the more natural way to work your heart, provides information about the kind of shape you are in, and may reproduce the symptoms you had that led to taking the stress test. Your doctor may choose to use medication to stress your heart if you are unable to walk briskly on a treadmill, have an abnormal EKG, or are unable to get your heart rate to the target level.

In addition to an EKG monitor, most stress tests today have some sort of imaging component (echocardiogram or nuclear myocardial perfusion imaging) to maximize the test's ability to detect coronary heart disease. Imaging the heart at the time of the stress test not only increases the test's accuracy but also provides useful secondary information about the heart's size, structure, and function.

There are three different types of traditional stress tests: the exercise treadmill test, the stress echocardiogram test, and the nuclear (myocardial perfusion imaging) test.

Exercise Treadmill Stress Test

An exercise treadmill test (ETT) is the most basic type of stress test. It's often referred to as a "plain vanilla" stress test because no imaging component is added to the test. Your heart rate, blood pressure, and EKG are monitored throughout a series of three-minute periods of advancing speed and grade on a standard motorized treadmill.

The exercise treadmill test is most useful if you have a low likelihood of heart disease and a normal baseline EKG. It is quick, safe, and inexpensive, but it is not all that reliable. Many medications and baseline EKG abnormalities commonly cause inaccurate stress test results.

Women, especially, often have inaccurate exercise treadmill test results. While ongoing studies are helping to decide the best type of stress test for women, experience makes me recommend that women avoid taking this test and go right to one of the imaging stress tests.

Advantages of the Exercise Treadmill Stress Test

- Quick, safe, and widely available
- Inexpensive

Disadvantages of the Exercise Treadmill Stress Test

- Patient must have a completely normal resting EKG
- Only 60 to 70 percent accurate, at best
- Often leads to additional, more definitive testing
- Women often have a "false positive" result

Echocardiogram Stress Test

A stress echocardiogram is a regular treadmill stress test that has an added imaging component. Ultrasound, or echocardiogram, pictures are taken of the heart at rest and immediately after the treadmill stress has been completed.

The main advantage of the stress echocardiogram is that it markedly improves your chances of detecting coronary heart disease (up to 70 to 85 percent) when compared to a treadmill stress test alone. In addition, the ultrasound pictures provide information about your heart's structure and function that regular treadmill tests can't provide. Stress echocardiograms provide a high degree of accuracy while offering safety and convenience at a reasonable cost to the patient.

Advantages of the Echocardiogram Stress Test

- Safe, noninvasive, and painless
- More accurate than treadmill testing alone
- Provides additional information about the size, structure, and function of the heart muscle
- Provides additional information about other heart structures, including the pericardium, the heart valves, and the aorta
- Stress can be induced by exercise or with medications, making the test more flexible than a routine exercise treadmill test

Disadvantages of the Echocardiogram Stress Test

- More costly than treadmill alone

- Still misses up to 15 to 20 percent of severe coronary artery disease in patients
- Imaging is limited in people with lung disease, large breasts, or obesity
- Requires technical expertise to obtain usable ultrasound images while the heart is maximally stressed

Nuclear (Myocardial Perfusion Imaging) Stress Test

A myocardial perfusion imaging stress test is a highly technical test that uses a small amount of a radioactive substance and a special camera to provide detailed pictures of the blood flow to the heart. Just as with a stress echocardiogram, the stress portion of a nuclear stress test can be done with a treadmill or with medication. The nuclear stress test is the most accurate type of stress test commonly performed today (see chapter 9 to read about new PET technology).

Immediately before and after exercise, a small, safe amount of a radioactive material is injected through an IV. This material circulates through the heart, allowing a special gamma camera to compare the radioactive activity of the heart before and after stress to detect areas of low blood flow caused by heart artery blockages.

Advantages of the Nuclear (Myocardial Perfusion Imaging) Stress Test

- Most accurate *commonly* performed stress test today
- Stress can be achieved with exercise or with medications
- Excellent at differentiating areas of old heart attacks and new areas of severely blocked arteries
- Helps predict future heart attacks and survival
- Excellent correlation with the heart angiogram, the gold standard in heart disease evaluation
- Provides information about the size and strength of the heart pump

Disadvantages of the Nuclear (Myocardial Perfusion Imaging) Stress Test

- Expensive
- Test takes two to four hours to complete

- Heavier patients require two separate days of testing
- Small amount of radioactive agent required
- Requires an IV
- Less accurate in patients who are obese or who have large breasts

What the Stress Test Can and *Can't* Tell You about Your Heart Health

There are a lot of good reasons to have a stress test, but if you take one you really need to know what your test results mean. You also need to know what they are not telling you.

What the Results of a Stress Test *Can* Tell You

Once your stress test is complete, your doctor will give you one of three results: the stress test was *normal*, *abnormal*, or *indeterminate*.

Normal Result

This result is great news. If it was chest pain that caused you to take the test, the result tells you that the pain you had was probably *not* due to blocked heart arteries. If you had chest pain prior to starting an exercise program, the result tells you that it's okay to start one and that no *major* heart blockages were found.

If you had a stress test to check if your heart disease treatment is being effective, then it tells you the treatment is working. Finally, if you had the stress test to screen for coronary heart disease, a normal reading tells you there were no severely blocked heart arteries.

Abnormal Result

An abnormal stress test result tells you one of two things: that you have *myocardial ischemia* or that you have had a *myocardial infarction*.

A stress test that shows an area of ischemia means that under resting conditions blood flow to the heart is normal, but that during the stress portion of the test the heart did not receive an adequate blood flow. Your heart loses adequate blood flow when at least one artery is blocked by more than about 70 percent.

Your stress test result also will be abnormal if dead heart muscle from an old heart attack is detected. A myocardial infarction, or heart attack, leaves an area of scar tissue in the heart muscle that never regains function. A stress test that shows an "*infarct*" means that at some time in the past a heart attack occurred but currently there are no new areas of the heart that are at risk.

Indeterminate Result

No test is perfect. Depending on the type of stress test you have, there is a 10 to 40 percent chance that the test will not be accurate or useful. If your stress test result is indeterminate, you will need to take a different type of stress test or undergo a more invasive heart catheterization to get the information you are looking for.

What the Results of a Stress Test *Can't* Tell You

Do you remember our friend Scott from the beginning of this chapter? Scott had a normal stress test and then went on to have a major heart attack just a few weeks later. Scott's wife wanted to know how that could have happened; you probably want to know as well.

The problem was not what the stress test told us about Scott's heart; the problem was what the stress test failed to tell us about Scott's heart.

The Stress Test's Dirty Little Secret

A stress test is not a great screening tool for coronary heart disease. In fact, when used alone it's a downright *terrible* screening tool for coronary heart disease.

Would you choose a cancer-screening test that could pick up only severe, advanced cancer? Of course not! The goal of a screening test is to detect the disease in its earliest stage, well before it can do you any significant harm.

Stress tests simply can't do that. They are frequently used for heart disease screening only because up until now it's all we've had. It's better than nothing but far from ideal.

Three factors limit the usefulness of the stress test as a screening tool:

1. Mild or moderate heart artery blockages (20 to 70 percent blocked) cause most heart attacks and sudden cardiac death.

2. Coronary artery disease does not cause any symptoms until an artery is more than 70 percent blocked.

3. Stress tests detect only severe (>70 percent) heart artery blockage.

It's always good news when you have a normal stress test result. However, it's important to remember what a stress test can and cannot tell you about your heart health. A normal stress test tells you that you have no *major blockages* in your heart arteries. A normal stress test tells you that the chest pain you've been having probably is not heart-related. And a normal stress test can help direct you toward a safe and effective exercise program. *A normal stress test result, however, tells you nothing about whether you have mild or moderate coronary artery disease and tells you very little about your risk of having a heart attack. Don't let a normal stress test give you a false sense of security about your heart.*

Summing It Up

Stress tests play a vital role in the evaluation, detection, and management of coronary heart disease. The stress test is the test of choice for evaluating heart-related symptoms such as chest pain, shortness of breath, and palpitations. Whether you take the test by exercising or with medication that mimics the effects of exercising, most stress tests will incorporate advanced imaging techniques such as ultrasound or nuclear imaging to maximize the chances of detecting coronary artery disease.

There are both upsides and downsides to stress tests. The pluses are that they are excellent in evaluating chest pain and evaluating the effectiveness of coronary heart disease treatment. The downside is that stress tests can detect only severe blockages in your heart arteries. They are limited in their ability to act as a screening tool for heart disease or in gauging your heart attack risk.

The stress test will continue to be used as part of the evaluation and prevention of coronary heart disease. Just remember that it needs to be used in conjunction with other tests and cardiac risk assessment tools to be valuable in predicting your cardiac risk.

Chapter 9

The Cutting Edge of Cardiology

Take Advantage of the Latest Imaging and
Stress Tests to Find Out Your Risk

The ideal way to know your cardiac risk is to know what's going on *inside* your heart arteries. Until now, doctors could make only an educated guess about what was happening inside your arteries based on your cardiac risk factors; now we have multiple options. Rapidly advancing technology now allows us to look inside your arteries to tell you exactly whether cholesterol plaque is building up inside them.

There are a number of exciting tests available today. In this chapter I will break them down into two categories: (1) screening tests to help determine your cardiac risk and (2) cutting-edge, one-stop, comprehensive cardiovascular evaluation tests.

Let's look at the more widely available screening tests first.

Screening Tests to Help Determine Your Cardiac Risk

These relatively inexpensive and widely available tests are valuable at providing extraordinary insight into your cardiac risk. They are most effective when used in combination with traditional and emerging cardiac risk factor assessment.

In general, these tests best serve patients who are at intermediate or moderate risk for coronary heart disease rather than those already known to be at the highest or lowest risk. When used properly these tests can better define your risk, diagnose coronary artery disease early, and help direct treatment.

The screening tests covered in this chapter include the heart scan, the carotid arteries intima-media thickness test, the brachial artery reactivity test, and the ankle-brachial index test.

The Heart Scan: Detecting Hardening of the Arteries

Do you know your calcium score?

If you don't, you may be missing out on one of the easiest ways to find out if you have coronary artery disease and to determine your risk for a heart attack. The heart scan is the first widely available, noninvasive, and affordable test that can look into your heart arteries to detect and quantify early atherosclerosis—*before* symptoms occur and *much earlier* than a stress test can detect it.

Let me tell you about the power of a heart scan and a patient I will never forget.

Tim is a forty-two-year-old father of five with no significant risk factors for heart disease. He is active, exercises regularly, and owns his own successful business. Tim came into my office wanting to know his risk for having a heart attack. In addition to giving him a routine physical examination, I had him have blood drawn for a fasting lipid panel.

Tim's lipid panel showed normal total and LDL cholesterol levels, but his HDL cholesterol was borderline at 39 mg/dL (normal is greater than 40 mg/dL). I thought about how aggressive I should be in treating it—Tim is only forty-two, and I didn't want to needlessly commit him to medications for the rest of his life.

Tim and I both wanted more information, so the next step was a heart scan.

We were shocked at the findings. Tim's calcium score was extremely high: he had a coronary artery calcium score of 350, which put him in the ninety-fifth percentile for men his age. That meant that he had more calcium building up in his arteries than ninety-five of every hundred men his age who take the test.

After flunking a stress test, Tim went on to have angioplasty and stents placed in two of his major heart arteries. He is now taking blood thinners as well as medications to raise his HDL and lower his LDL cholesterol levels.

The heart scan definitely saved Tim's life.

What Is a Heart Scan?

The heart scan is a special type of X-ray that uses technology called electron beam computed tomography (EBCT or EBT). It is a screening test used for the early detection of heart disease that could lead to a heart attack. Heart scans are unique because they can discover atherosclerosis long before symptoms develop and earlier than a stress test can find it.

Heart scans work by detecting and measuring calcium deposits in your heart arteries. *Normal coronary arteries have no detectable cholesterol or calcium. Ever.* But as atherosclerosis and cholesterol invade coronary arteries, calcium deposits invade the artery over time. These bright, reflective calcium deposits can easily be detected and quantified with a heart scan.

The heart scan procedure is extremely fast and simple and does not require any special preparation. You don't even need an IV inserted to have the test. Having a heart scan is similar to having a CT scan or a simple X-ray.

During the heart scan, you need to lie flat and really hold still for about a minute while the ultrafast camera scans your chest; you need to hold your breath during the imaging, to limit any motion. But that's the whole test. It couldn't be much easier.

Heart Scan Advantages

- Takes only a few minutes to complete
- No pain, needles, poking, or prodding
- No special preparations (such as fasting)
- No significant side effects
- Detects heart disease *before* symptoms develop and *earlier* than a stress test
- Accurate and reproducible test results
- Proven incremental benefit in predicting risk over risk factor evaluation alone

---

Calcium Scores and What They Mean

Heart scan information is compiled by a computer and interpreted by a cardiologist. The results are given as a *coronary artery calcium (CAC) score*, showing how much calcium has built up in your arteries.

To help you gauge your risk, your CAC score is given in two different ways: as a *total calcium score* and as an *age-based calcium score*. This gives you the big picture in assessing your risk, which many experts label as your *plaque burden*. Your plaque burden is an excellent predictor of your heart attack risk.

Total Coronary Artery Calcium Score

Dr. Arthur Agatston, author of *The South Beach Diet*, is responsible for the most commonly used heart scan scoring system, the CAC score. This score measures the volume, density, and distribution of calcium in the coronary arteries, which shows up as specks of white on a heart scan. The CAC score is a sum of all the specks of calcium that are detected through-out the heart arteries.

To determine the total coronary artery calcium score, a computer assigns a number to each speck of calcium that's detected. Simply put, if there is no calcium in the arteries, the score is 0. If there are fifty specks, the score is 50. The more calcium the computer detects, the higher your score. The list below shows the CAC categories and the related coronary heart disease risk.

Coronary artery calcium score and accompanying cardiac risk

- 0 indicates no calcium buildup: extremely low risk.
- 1 to 10 indicates minimal plaque buildup: very low risk.
- 11 to 100 indicates mild plaque buildup: intermediate risk.
- 101 to 400 indicates moderate plaque buildup: high risk.
- More than 400 indicates extensive plaque buildup: very high risk.

Age-Based Percentile Score

The second way to interpret a heart scan test result is to compare your score with other people of your age and gender. This gives you an age-based percentile score. For example, a CAC score of 100 in a sixty-year-old man puts him in the fiftieth percentile for risk, but a CAC score of 100 in a forty-year-old would put that person closer to the ninetieth percentile rank—most forty-year-olds are not going to have that much calcium built up already. Using this method of scoring, the higher your rank compared to other people of the same age and sex, the higher your risk for complications from heart disease in the future.

Are Heart Scans Safe?

Heart scans are extremely safe. However, there are three types of risks in using them that you need to be aware of: the risk of radiation exposure, the risk of the heart scan triggering a series of unnecessary cardiovascular tests, and the risk of the heart scan missing potentially dangerous "soft" cholesterol plaque.

Being Exposed to Radiation

A small amount of radiation exposure is the primary medical risk associated with heart scans. The radiation you receive from a scan is equivalent to what you receive from having three chest X-rays or one mammogram. This amount of radiation is well within the radiation safety guidelines for the amount of medical radiation it is considered safe to receive in a year. If you have no other major radiation exposure in a year, the radiation from a heart scan is considered negligible.

Having Unnecessary Medical Testing

Another risk of heart scans is that they can lead to a series of unnecessary medical tests. That's because it is possible to have a significantly abnormal heart scan and still have no *clinically significant* heart blockage. If a heart scan is severely abnormal, that often leads to further evaluation with a stress test. The stress test has a 10 to 30 percent chance that its result will be abnormal or indeterminate, and that can lead to more invasive tests, such as a cardiac angiogram.

Additional medical testing following a heart scan is one of the big concerns of insurance companies and professionals who manage health care costs for entire populations such as the government.

Missing Hidden "Soft" Cholesterol Plaque

No test is perfect. The downfall of the heart scan is that it can't detect *soft plaque*. That's what cholesterol plaque is called if it doesn't contain any calcium—some plaques, especially newer ones, may not yet contain calcium. While calcium that has invaded cholesterol plaque—making it "hard"—will show up as a light speck on the heart scan, if there is no calcium in the plaque the heart scan will not detect the plaque. Therefore it's controversial that people under age forty have a heart scan, because younger people usually don't have any buildup of calcium yet in their arteries.

Should You Have a Heart Scan?

When used indiscriminately, the heart scan can be a giant waste of money and lead you on a wild goose chase of cardiovascular testing. However, when it's used correctly, the heart scan can be one of the most useful heart tests you will ever have, and it could help save your life.

Let me share the story of another of my patients whose heart scan probably saved her life.

Leslie was fifty-one years old when we met in my office. She had come for a second opinion regarding her cholesterol level. For years her doctor had been telling her that her cholesterol was borderline and to increase her exercise and watch her diet. She wanted to know if borderline was good enough or if she needed medications to bring her cholesterol lower.

I explained to Leslie that cholesterol affects everyone differently. Some people with a borderline cholesterol level go on to develop significant heart problems, but some don't. We needed additional information to tip the scales in the direction of either being more aggressive with medications to lower her cholesterol or to continue diet and lifestyle treatment (which really wasn't doing much to bring her cholesterol down).

To get the information I needed, Leslie had a heart scan. The result of her test was only mildly abnormal, but that was all I needed to know. Indeed, Leslie had evidence of calcium in her heart arteries, which meant that cholesterol and plaque were already building up. While her short-term risk of a heart attack was small, her risk for problems down the road was at least moderate. I felt very confident starting Leslie on a cholesterol-lowering drug and an aspirin a day. Her cholesterol level came down, and she has been great ever since.

Both Leslie and my patient Tim, whom I mentioned earlier, had their lives saved by their heart scans. Tim's story was more dramatic: his heart scan showed that he needed urgent, immediate treatment to reduce his risk of a heart attack and sudden cardiac death. Leslie's story was less dramatic, but it's one I hear often. She would have been in no danger during the next few years, but if we had left her borderline cholesterol level untreated, cholesterol would have continued to attack her arteries and led to heart problems down the road.

Patients Unlikely to Benefit from a Heart Scan

I do not recommend heart scans for young people or for people at either end of the cardiovascular risk scale.

First, you shouldn't bother with one if you're young. Heart scans are not recommended for people younger than forty, because even if you have early atherosclerosis you may not have any calcium develop until about forty.

Second, if you are at either end of the cardiac risk spectrum, you probably will not substantially benefit from having a heart scan. If you don't have any cardiac risk factors (either traditional or emerging) you are extremely unlikely to develop coronary artery disease, so a heart scan will likely add nothing to your overall risk assessment.

At the other end of the risk spectrum—you have diabetes, multiple cardiac risk factors, or known coronary artery disease—you are already known to be at high risk for coronary artery disease, and a heart scan, no matter what the results, will not change that fact.

Patients Likely to Benefit from a Heart Scan

Heart scans are most useful for patients who have a medium risk of coronary heart disease based on either traditional or emerging cardiac risk factors. So you might want to think of the heart scan as a risk-factor tiebreaker. If you fall in the middle of high and low risk for heart complications, having a heart scan can reclassify you to either the high-risk or the low-risk group.

For example, if you are a medium-risk patient based on traditional cardiac risk factors but have an abnormal heart scan, you are moved up to the high-risk category and treated accordingly. If you are a medium-risk patient with a completely normal heart scan, you *may* be able to take a more conservative approach to managing your heart risk, relying on lifestyle changes rather than prescription medications (just don't forget about the heart scan's inability to detect soft plaque).

Typical Patients Who Benefit from a Heart Scan

- Fifty-two-year-old with high blood pressure and a borderline cholesterol level
- Forty-eight-year-old with a mildly elevated cholesterol level who is reluctant to start or noncompliant with cholesterol-lowering medications
- Forty-three-year-old with a strong family history for heart disease who wants to know her risk for having a heart attack
- Forty-year-old whose father died at forty-five and whose uncle developed heart disease in his forties

Heart Scans Guide Your Cholesterol Treatment

Determining your ideal cholesterol goal is another great reason to have a heart scan. Remember, all LDL cholesterol goals are based on how many risk factors you have for heart disease. The higher your risk, the lower you should target your LDL cholesterol level.

An abnormal heart scan result can make a huge difference in what your target LDL cholesterol should be. Most moderate-risk patients have an LDL cholesterol goal of less than 130 mg/dL. An abnormal heart scan, however, pushes your LDL cholesterol goal down to less than 100 mg/dL and maybe even to less than 70 mg/dL.

Will Insurance Pay for a Heart Scan?

Insurance companies don't often pay for "screening" tests. At this point in time you should assume that you will have to pay for the test out of your own pocket. Some health plans are starting to cover all or at least some of the expense, but even if you're partially reimbursed for the test, you still pay out of pocket and then submit the bill to your insurance company for reimbursement.

Expect to pay $400 to $600 for your heart scan; the test price varies, but in general the price is coming down quickly. My advice is to look for specials or package deals. A massive increase in the number of heart scan centers has produced a competitive market as well as price wars. Many centers will offer to scan other parts of your body as part of the heart scan cost or will provide whole-body scans at reduced rates.

The Bottom Line

The heart scan uses the newest X-ray technology to detect calcium that has built up in your heart arteries. Calcium in the arteries means they are being attacked by atherosclerosis.

Heart scans can make a huge impact in your fight against coronary heart disease. They detect coronary artery disease and atherosclerosis before symptoms develop and earlier than a stress test ever could.

For people at moderate risk for coronary heart disease based on traditional and emerging risk factors, the heart scan is an excellent tool to define their risk and to help target their cholesterol level goal.

The Carotid Arteries Intima-Media Thickness Test

Atherosclerosis is an equal opportunity opponent: it attacks all the arteries in the body, not just your heart arteries. If cholesterol plaque and atherosclerosis are anywhere in your body, you are at increased risk for cardiac problems.

One way to determine if you have atherosclerosis is, of course, to evaluate your heart arteries. But heart arteries are challenging to check because they are small, deep in the chest, and continually move with each heartbeat. The carotid arteries in the neck, on the other hand, are very easy to evaluate because they are larger, lie right beneath the skin, and are relatively motionless. The carotid arteries intima-media thickness (IMT) test looks at your carotid arteries, which gives us a good idea as to what is happening in your heart arteries.

The two carotid arteries, one on each side of the neck, are the critical pipelines of blood to the brain and to the face. The left and right common carotid arteries branch into an internal carotid artery and an external carotid artery. Though the carotid arteries are most often associated with strokes, not heart attacks, they actually act as windows to the heart arteries. Whatever is going on inside the carotid arteries tends to mirror what is going on in the coronary arteries.

How Does the Carotid IMT Work?

The carotid IMT uses ultrasound to evaluate the thickness of the inner (intima) and middle (media) layers of the carotid arteries as a predictor of the presence of coronary artery disease. Studies have proven that the thicker the intima-media, the higher the risk for heart attack and stroke; studies also have proven that the carotid IMT measurement is an accurate predictor of the presence of coronary heart disease and that carotid artery cholesterol buildup is an independent risk factor for heart attacks and stroke.

The test works likes this. All arteries in the body are composed of three layers: the inner or intima layer, the middle or media layer, and the outer or adventia layer. The intima, composed of endothelial cells that play a pivotal role in the development of atherosclerosis, is the prime target for invading cholesterol. If the endothelium becomes damaged or dysfunctional, LDL cholesterol can then attack it, beginning a dangerous buildup of cholesterol plaque.

If the LDL continues its invasion and cholesterol plaque continues to build, the carotid intima-media become thicker and thicker. The ultrasound waves detect and measure the buildup and provide a risk evaluation based on its thickness. For every 0.1 mm increase in intima-media thickness, the relative risk of coronary heart disease increases by more than 10 percent.

Having the Test

Ultrasound is a technology commonly used in several types of medical practice, from obstetrics and gynecology to vascular and cardiology. The technology works by having a small probe send and receive high-frequency ultrasound waves. The waves bounce off objects in the body and return to the receiver in distinctive forms, depending on the size, shape, and composition of what they bounce off. The waves that were generated are then converted into two-dimensional pictures for doctors to review.

The carotid IMT test may be done in your doctor's office or in a hospital. The test requires no fasting or special preparation, and no IV or contrast is needed. The test does not use any ionizing radiation, so it can be done as often as needed to follow treatment progress.

Trained ultrasound sonographers perform the IMT test, which takes about thirty minutes to complete. The technician simply rubs some imaging gel on your neck and then gently moves the ultrasound probe back and forth over each side of the neck to obtain images.

Should You Have a Carotid IMT Test?

The same factors to decide if you should have a heart scan also apply to whether you should have a carotid IMT test. If you already know that you are at very low risk (you have no cardiac risk factors) or at very high risk (you have a history of heart attack or angioplasty), you will not substantially benefit from a carotid IMT test.

If you are at moderate risk for coronary heart disease (you have at least one cardiovascular risk factor), you will benefit from knowing whether you have atherosclerosis in your arteries. Identifying cholesterol buildup in your arteries is important because it may dramatically change your treatment and your prognosis.

The Bottom Line

Carotid artery IMT measurements provide a safe, inexpensive, reproducible, and accurate assessment of your arterial health. Knowing the thickness of the carotid intima-media gives you an excellent gauge of whether you have atherosclerosis and/or coronary artery disease and, when taken in conjunction with cholesterol levels and general cardiac risk, can be a powerful predictor of heart attack and stroke risk. Just like the heart scans, it is also a great way to help decide how aggressive you need to be with lowering your cholesterol levels.

The Brachial Artery Reactivity Test

Most of the tests used to assess risk for coronary heart disease rely on imaging the arteries to visualize the cholesterol plaque. The earliest evidence that arteries are being attacked by cholesterol, however, comes not from the way they *look* but from the way they *behave*.

The brachial artery reactivity test (BART) is an indirect way to assess artery damage and the risk for coronary heart disease. Just as with the carotid arteries, any damage done to the brachial artery signifies similar damage or dysfunction in the heart's coronary arteries.

If you want to detect the first signs that your arteries are being damaged, then the brachial artery reactivity test is for you. No test can detect damaged arteries earlier.

How Does BART Work?

A healthy inner layer of your arterial wall is the cornerstone to preventing atherosclerosis. As you read earlier, the innermost layer of your heart artery is called the intima, and it is lined with a thin layer of endothelial cells, called the endothelium.

A healthy endothelium produces a substance called nitric oxide, which protects the artery from LDL cholesterol attack. It can do this by preventing inflammation in the area, preventing local clotting, and causing dilation of the blood vessels to allow extra blood through when needed. When the endothelium becomes damaged or dysfunctional, it decreases its production of nitric oxide, and many of these protective properties stop working, allowing cholesterol to attack and atherosclerosis to begin.

One of the best ways to evaluate the health and function of the endothelium is to measure the *flow-mediated vasodilator response*—in other words, test to see how well the artery responds to stress by how much it dilates and how much blood flow increases through the vessel.

Normal arteries dilate in response to stress and cause a large increase in blood flow. Abnormal or dysfunctional arteries constrict in response to stress, allowing only a small increase in blood flow or none at all.

An abnormal brachial artery response to stress correlates well with coronary heart disease and an increased risk of heart-related events.

Having the BART Test

The BART test is available only in some cardiologists' offices and in special heart disease prevention clinics. The test is very safe, inexpensive, and

> ### *Factors That Damage Your Endothelium*
>
> - High levels of LDL cholesterol
> - Low levels of HDL cholesterol
> - Smoke toxins
> - Infectious agents
> - High blood sugar (diabetes mellitus)
> - High homocysteine levels
> - High blood pressure

painless. There is no need for an IV, and no contrast or radiation is involved. The test takes only twenty to thirty minutes to complete.

Before you take the test, you need to fast for twelve hours and be sure to avoid caffeine, smoking, and other stimulants. When the test begins, a technician places a blood pressure cuff on your arm above your elbow, over your brachial artery, which is the artery that supplies the arm with blood. The blood pressure cuff is then *overinflated* to about 50 mm Hg over your resting top (systolic) blood pressure. The cuff is left inflated for five minutes to create stress to the artery wall.

Normal vs. Abnormal BART Test Results

When the cuff is deflated, the normal brachial artery dilates, allowing a sixfold increase in blood flow through the artery. An abnormal test result occurs when a dysfunctional artery is not able to dilate (and may even constrict or narrow), causing a limited or decreased blood flow response to stress. Instead of the normal sixfold increase in blood flow, a dysfunctional artery may allow only a twofold increase in flow or even no change in flow.

Should You Have a BART Test?

The brachial artery reactivity test has a unique niche in the evaluation of coronary heart disease risk: it detects the earliest signs of atherosclerosis. The BART test is especially useful for younger patients (under age forty), who likely do not yet have enough cholesterol built up or calcium deposited for it to be detected by other imaging modalities, such as the heart scan or stress test.

Let's look at how BART is commonly utilized.

Laura is the thirty-seven-year-old wife of a cardiologist specializing in heart disease prevention. Despite her heart-healthy lifestyle—she was at her ideal weight, ate a healthy diet, and loved to hike, ski, and snowshoe—she developed a high LDL cholesterol level. She didn't have much room to improve her diet or exercise, but she buckled down even harder by increasing her exercise and cutting out snacks. Unfortunately, her bad cholesterol remained elevated, at 165 mg/dL.

The dilemma Laura and her husband faced was this: should an otherwise healthy, active young woman with elevated LDL cholesterol be started on cholesterol medication?

Before they jumped into drug treatment, Laura and her cardiologist husband wanted more information. They already knew that Laura's short-term risk for a heart attack was low, but they wanted to know if her elevated bad cholesterol was setting her up for damage down the road.

Neither stress testing nor a heart scan would be useful for Laura. Stress tests detect only severe, advanced disease (which she clearly did not have), and heart scans rely on detecting calcium infiltrating an atherosclerotic plaque, which usually doesn't show up until about age forty, or even later in women.

They turned to the BART test.

Since BART gives us evidence as to whether endothelial dysfunction, the absolute earliest step in atherosclerosis, is taking place, Laura could find out if her elevated LDL cholesterol was causing endothelial dysfunction. If that was the case, then Laura and her husband would feel more comfortable treating her high cholesterol with medication. If it turned out that the endothelium was normal, they would continue lifestyle changes and hold off on medication.

Laura passed the brachial artery reactivity test with flying colors: her arteries showed no evidence of early damage. Armed with this knowledge, she elected not to start cholesterol medication and planned to follow up with a yearly BART test. When and if the test becomes abnormal, she'll start taking medication.

The Bottom Line

A simple brachial artery reactivity test can identify a healthy artery versus one that is damaged by the earliest effects of atherosclerosis. It is often used as a tiebreaker when trying to decide whether low or borderline cholesterol levels should be attacked with medication.

The Ankle-Brachial Index Test

Some of you may be asking at this point, "Are all the techniques used to measure my cardiac risk high-tech and expensive?" The answer is no, though the ones that give the most information tend to be the most expensive.

The ankle-brachial index test, or ABI, is what I call the "poor man's" tool for additional cardiac risk information. The ankle-brachial index test can help detect peripheral vascular disease, which, just like carotid plaque and endothelial dysfunction, correlates well with the presence of coronary artery disease.

The ABI is not an imaging technique, nor does it screen for early plaque formation. It is the ratio of the systolic blood pressure taken at the ankle divided by the systolic blood pressure in the arm. An ABI of 0.90 or less is considered abnormal and correlates with moderate to severe atherosclerosis in the leg arteries.

This inexpensive, painless, and easy-to-perform test may be useful to determine your cardiac and vascular risk when used in conjunction with cholesterol levels and a total cardiac risk assessment.

Cutting-Edge, One-Stop, Comprehensive Cardiovascular Evaluation Tests

This second group of high-tech testing takes cardiovascular evaluation to an entirely new level. These tests are the future of cardiology and heart disease prevention.

The three tests this section covers include cardiac MRI, cardiac CT, and PET stress testing. While I think it's important for you to know about this rapidly evolving technology, be aware that all of these tests are not yet widely available. Use of cardiac CT and cardiac PET scanners is expanding quickly. There are already nearly a hundred of the newest, most advanced cardiac CT scanners in the United States, and the numbers are exploding rapidly. The massive size and expense of cardiac MRI cameras currently limit their availability primarily to universities and academic medical centers.

This state-of-the-art and rapidly advancing technology will, without a doubt, change the way we detect, treat, and prevent coronary heart disease forever. As costs come down and reimbursement issues settle out, you will begin to hear much more.

Let's start your high-tech tour by looking at cardiac MRI.

Cardiac MRI: Opening a Window to the Heart

The MRI has been used for years to image all areas of the body. Only relatively recently, however, has there been much focus on the heart. The cardiac MRI is a unique heart-imaging tool that, unlike all other cardiac imaging tests, does not use X-rays or ultrasound. The cardiac MRI uses a strong magnetic field and radio waves to create viewable 3-D images. While it takes somewhat of a physics lesson to understand how the MRI works, it's interesting to know a few basic points about the test that is pushing the boundaries of heart disease detection and evaluation.

Here's how it works: Water molecules (H_2O) are present in every tissue in the body. Hydrogen atoms are present in water molecules (the "H" in H_2O). The proton (positively charged atom) in the inner core of the hydrogen atom vibrates when bombarded with bursts of "magnetic" energy. Vibrating protons then emit radio-frequency energy. Various tissues emit slightly different radio-frequency energies, differentiating tissues that are adjacent to each other. The MRI "camera" detects this radio-frequency energy and converts it to a viewable 3-D image. The 3-D image can be viewed whole or "sliced" like a loaf of bread to see great detail in any part of the image.

The images from most cardiac MRI images are significantly improved with the addition of a contrast agent. This agent, called gadolinium, is not ionic-based, making it much easier and safer to use than contrasts used in other imaging modalities, including cardiac angiograms and even CT angiography.

Evaluating Coronary Artery Disease

The cardiac MRI is truly a one-stop shop for the detection and evaluation of *all aspects* of coronary artery disease. Not only can it look for and find coronary artery disease, but it also can differentiate stable from unstable plaque formation, determine relative myocardial blood flow (like a stress test), and differentiate live heart muscle from dead heart muscle (so-called myocardial viability).

Visualizing Small Vessels

The coronary arteries are only 3 to 4 mm wide at their largest points. Being able to visualize these small internal vessels with a noninvasive imaging test is quite remarkable, and it has not been possible until now. Now we no longer have to rely on invasive angiogram procedures to look for blockages in the heart arteries.

Distinguishing between Stable and Unstable Plaque

All coronary artery blockages are not created equally. The difference between life and death often comes down to whether your blockage is due to a stable or an unstable plaque. A stable 70 percent plaque may never cause you problems, while an unstable 30 percent plaque may rupture, causing a heart attack or sudden cardiac death.

The cardiac MRI not only can detect coronary artery blockage but also can differentiate dangerous, unstable plaque from stable plaque. Knowing which kind of plaque exists in your arteries could be life-saving.

Determining Myocardial Perfusion

Treating coronary artery disease can get a little tricky. It takes more information than just how much of the artery is clogged to determine whether the patient needs a surgical procedure or just medical treatment.

It's all about the blood flow to the heart, which is why stress tests can be so important—they evaluate your heart's blood flow, or myocardial perfusion, in response to exercise.

We can now perform a cardiac stress test at the same time as the cardiac MRI, enabling doctors to differentiate hemodynamically significant blockages that need invasive treatment from less significant lesions that just require medical therapy.

Detecting Myocardial Viability

When part of the heart muscle goes without adequate blood supply because of blocked heart arteries, it begins to protect itself by going into "hibernation." During hibernation, myocardial cells turn things down really low, use very little oxygen, and don't work that hard. The cells are still alive, or have *myocardial viability*, and if they can regain their blood supply they will recover complete function.

Detecting hibernating cells is an important but difficult job. Until now, stress tests have been the best way to look for hibernating myocardium, but now cardiac MRI may be the approach of the future.

New studies have shown that the cardiac MRI can tell the difference between dead and hibernating heart cells to help guide your treatment.

Quantifying Heart Function

Once an area of the heart dies, it can never regain its function. So the larger the area involved in a heart attack, the weaker the heart becomes and the worse is the prognosis. The cardiac MRI can detect and quantify the amount and severity of dead heart tissue and can determine the overall function of the heart muscle.

The Bottom Line

The cardiac MRI has the potential to be an incredibly useful one-stop supertest to win the war against coronary heart disease.

Cardiac MRI Benefits

- Provides detailed 3-D images of the heart and other vascular structures
- Does not expose patient to radiation or radioactive isotopes
- Is painless and noninvasive, requiring only an IV for contrast injection
- Test takes only fifteen to forty-five minutes
- Images not limited by bone, lungs, fat, or breast tissue
- Detects coronary artery disease in earliest stages
- Detects heart attack risk by differentiating between stable and unstable plaque
- Can perform a stress test and coronary imaging at the same time
- Images valves and heart size, shape, and dimensions
- Detects areas of old heart attacks and scar tissue
- Movies can be obtained of valve and heart muscle structure and function

Cardiac MRI Risks and Downsides

- Medications required to slow heart rate down for coronary imaging
- Metallic objects and pacemakers or internal defibrillators limit some patients from having test

- Some patients experience claustrophobia in the MRI scanner
- Currently not widely available
- Costly equipment
- Not all cardiac imaging covered by insurance

Should You Have a Cardiac MRI?

At this time, a cardiac MRI is not for everyone. The device's advanced technology comes at a high cost both to own and to operate, and specialized technicians and physician training are needed to use it. While the cost is coming down, all of these factors currently limit its widespread use and availability. The cardiac MRI may become the ultimate one-stop heart test, so don't be surprised if within the next three to five years you see a cardiac MRI coming to an office near you.

Cardiac CT (Computed Tomography)

Before looking at the cardiac CT, read the following "dream" scenario:

Eric is a forty-four-year-old tax attorney and father of two. He is twenty pounds overweight, a former smoker, and has high blood pressure controlled with medication. He has not exercised in two years but is interested in starting an exercise program to get back into shape. Eric wants to know if it's safe to start exercising, and he wants to know his risk of developing coronary heart disease.

Eric goes to the cardiologists' office to have a revolutionary heart test. He stays in his street clothes and has an IV placed in his arm. He lies down on the imaging table and holds his breath while dye is injected and a series of images are obtained. Thirty-five seconds later the images are completed. Eric then gets a three-minute infusion of a medication to "stress" his heart followed by another thirty-five seconds of imaging. After a total of just a few minutes Eric's test is finished. The IV comes out and he goes home.

The next day his cardiologist calls to give him his test results. Eric had had two areas of soft, unstable plaque buildup in his coronary arteries—one was a 20 percent blockage and one was a 35 percent blockage. He also had one stable, calcified coronary artery blockage of 35 percent. His coronary artery calcium score was 145, putting him in the ninetieth percentile for men his age. The stress test portion of his study was normal, proving that there were no high-grade blockages in his arteries. His heart chambers were normal in size and the pump function of his heart was normal.

Eric was surprised to learn that he already had developed coronary artery disease. He was thankful and excited to have the opportunity to identify and treat it early, before it caused problems. Eric's doctor started him on a new cholesterol medication to lower his bad cholesterol and raise his good cholesterol. In addition, he was given a blood thinner and was told to repeat the test in two to three years. Eric started exercising the next day.

In this scenario, Eric had the ultimate, one-stop noninvasive heart test. This test is an absolute dream come true for both doctors and patients, telling you everything you need to know about your heart. Until now you would have needed an echocardiogram, a stress test, a heart scan, and an invasive cardiac angiogram to get the same information. Now it can all be done in just a few minutes with a single amazing test.

You may think that this dream test is just that, a dream, but Eric's test isn't some high-tech fantasy; this test is available today! Eric had a cardiac PET/CT angiography test, also known as cardiac CT or cardiac multidetector computed tomography (MDCT). Cardiac MDCT is a breakthrough, noninvasive imaging technology used to evaluate the coronary arteries for blockages, calcification, and blood flow. This exciting new tool is opening up doors to the early detection and prevention of coronary heart disease.

What Is Computed Tomography (CT)?

CT scans (commonly called "CAT" scans) are a specialized form of X-ray exam. They provide very detailed two-dimensional images of body structures, then "slice" the images into pieces for easy viewing and interpretation.

CT scans have been around for thirty years and are routinely used for the evaluation of multiple medical problems. Specialists including gastroenterologists, neurologists, pulmonologists, orthopedists, and oncologists utilize CT scans every day in their practices; in fact, up until now, cardiologists were about the only specialists who didn't rely on CT scans for the regular assessment of their patients. This kind of scan was not very useful for evaluating coronary artery disease because it didn't provide enough resolution to see the small heart arteries clearly. In addition, the CT scan took pictures too slowly to capture clear movie-type images of the moving blood and heart arteries.

All that has changed.

Multidetector CT: High-Speed and High-Tech

You probably know what it's like to try to take a picture of a moving object with the wrong camera speed; all you see is a blur. The same holds true for imaging the heart. Advanced imaging techniques with a strong emphasis on speed now allow us to clearly image the moving heart arteries.

One of the keys to improving the CT scan's ability to take clear moving images was adding more image detectors. Initially the device had just one detector, then two, then four; now there are sixty-four detectors and counting. The more detectors you have, the clearer the image of the beating heart. And not only do more detectors provide a clearer image of the heart, they also provide three-dimensional pictures and movies of the beating heart.

The CT is now ready for prime-time use in the detection of coronary heart disease. There are now close to a hundred heart centers across the United States utilizing the power of cardiac MDCT, and that number is expected to double over the next eighteen months.

CT Angiography and Calcium Scoring

Two basic methods of cardiac scanning are performed with the new and improved MDCT: CT angiography and calcium scoring.

CT Angiography

The heart catheterization (or coronary angiogram) is considered the current gold standard for evaluating the heart arteries. Its invasive nature and long list of potential complications, however, limit its use for the routine evaluation of coronary artery disease.

We now have a solution to that problem. CT angiography is a *non-invasive* heart catheterization. It provides beautifully detailed images of the heart arteries, cholesterol blockage, coronary stents, and bypass grafts without most of the troublesome complications of a traditional catheterization.

The CT angiography test requires only an IV and can be done in ten to thirty minutes (even in less time with the newest cameras). No hospitalization is required, and no invasive catheters are needed. The test not only provides a complete evaluation of the coronary arteries but also defines the size and structure of the heart and provides the coronary artery calcium score (see below).

In addition to heart-related imaging, CT angiography is excellent for evaluating issues in the brain, including cancer and cerebral aneurysms, as well as the carotid arteries, the aorta, the renal arteries, and pelvic and leg vessels.

Calcium Scoring

Calcium scoring visualizes atherosclerotic changes in the coronary arteries. A person with no symptoms of coronary disease but with a calcium score in the eightieth percentile has fifteen times the relative risk of cardiac events compared to an individual without coronary calcium. If no calcium is detected, the risk of cardiac events is close to zero. Calcium scoring is discussed in detail in the heart scan section.

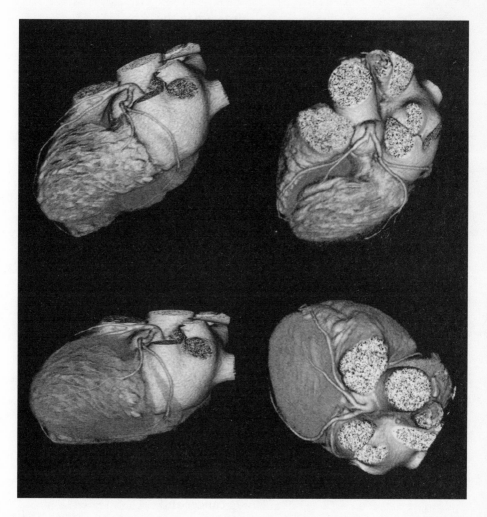

State-of-the-art 64-slice CT angiography showing detailed images of the coronary arteries, heart and major vessels. *Courtesy of Toshiba America Medical Systems*

Combining Cardiac CT with PET Stress Testing

Cardiac MDCT provides a wealth of information about your heart and your heart arteries. Now we have taken even that test to the next level. The newest stress test technology (known as a PET scan) has been added to the cardiac CT scan to create a cardiac "supertest."

Mark Nathan, M.D., F.A.C.C., is a nuclear cardiologist and pioneer in this field. Dr. Nathan is responsible for bringing the first cardiac

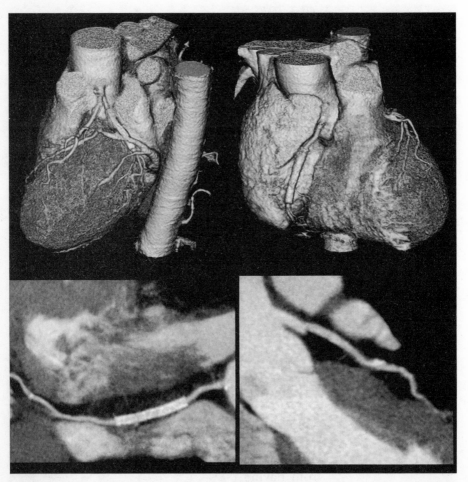

Amazingly detailed 64-slice CT angiography showing a coronary stent placed inside a heart artery blockage. *Courtesy of Toshiba America Medical Systems*

PET/CT combined scanner to northern California and is amazed at the results. He says,

"Combining the detailed images of the heart and arteries from the CT scan and fusing it with the latest stress test technology from the PET scan is like a dream come true! In one complete, quick, safe, noninvasive test I can confidently tell my patients how much cholesterol plaque they have building up in their arteries, the functional significance of any heart artery blockage, as well as important information about their heart size and function."

He goes on to say, "There is no doubt in my mind that this is just the tip of the iceberg. High-tech cardiac imaging is here to stay and it's going to change the way future generations detect, treat, and prevent heart disease."

Positron emission tomography (PET) is the newest type of stress test that takes advantage of a stronger and even faster-acting radioactive substance (rubidium) to evaluate the blood flow to the heart. PET stress testing has a number of advantages over the traditional "nuclear" stress test. It takes less time to have the test, it is more accurate, and best of all it can easily and safely be combined with a cardiac CT to provide a comprehensive evaluation of your overall heart health.

Summing It Up

New technology is changing the way we attack coronary heart disease. There are two general classifications of new cardiac tests: those that are general screening tests to help gauge cardiac risk, and those more expensive, ultra-high-tech tests that will probably become the one-stop cardiac test of the future.

Heart scans, carotid arteries intima-media thickness tests, and the brachial arterial reactivity test are all screening tests that may be useful components in the evaluation of coronary artery disease. They are best employed in combination with cholesterol testing and routine risk factor analysis in determining your overall heart risk.

Cardiac MRI and cardiac CT, with or without the addition of PET technology, no doubt represent the future of cardiology and the future of coronary artery disease detection and prevention. These ultra-high-tech tests are available in some locations now, and their use is expanding rapidly. We are not far from having one of these tests break through to become the ultimate noninvasive, one-stop heart test to tell us almost everything we need to know about your heart and your risk.

STEP FOUR

Putting It All Together: What's Your Risk?

I know we have covered a lot of ground thus far, but we are coming down the homestretch. Now it's time to put together all the information we learned in Steps One to Three before we bring it home in Step Five, with a detailed Heart Smart treatment plan.

In this section, we'll start out your cardiac risk assessment by checking a fasting lipoprotein profile. Remember, LDL cholesterol is your primary treatment target for preventing and treating coronary heart disease. Then we'll go through, identify, and add up how many traditional cardiac risk factors you have. I then provide you with what to look for with some of the more important emerging cardiac risk factors and tests that can help gauge your risk.

Once this step is accomplished, there are two different ways that you can put it all together to determine your cardiac risk. One way is to use a risk scale adopted from the National Cholesterol Education Programs (NCEP) risk assessment guide. I have modified the NCEP guide by adding risk assessment information based on newer emerging cardiac risk factors and new testing, such as the heart scan. *Heart Smart* is the only source where you can find this cutting-edge information.

The other available risk assessment tool is based on the Framingham Heart Study. This risk assessment tool utilizes a simple questionnaire to give you points based on your cardiac risk factors. The more points you have, the higher your ten-year risk of developing coronary heart disease and heart attacks.

Both approaches are accurate and up-to-date ways to find out your cardiac risk.

Good luck!

Chapter 10

Cardiac Risk Assessment Tools

Cardiac Risk Assessment Based on the National Cholesterol Education Program

Check your cholesterol

Step 1: You can't go too far in assessing your cardiac risk without knowing your cholesterol numbers. Don't be fooled by total cholesterol levels. All treatment guidelines are based on LDL and HDL cholesterol as well as on triglyceride levels. LDL cholesterol is your first and primary treatment target. The test you need is the fasting complete lipoprotein profile.

LDL Cholesterol—Primary Target of Therapy

<70 mg/dL	New high-risk target
<100 mg/dL	Optimal
100–129 mg/dL	Above optimal
130–159 mg/dL	Borderline high
160–189 mg/dL	High
>189 mg/dL	Very high

HDL Cholesterol—Higher Is Better

<40 mg/dL	Low
>60 mg/dL	Optimal

Triglycerides—Target after Treating LDL Cholesterol

<150 mg/dL	Normal
150–199 mg/dL	Borderline high
200–499 mg/dL	High
>499 mg/dL	Very high

Determine other traditonal risk factors

Step 2: Now that you know *all your cholesterol numbers*, turn your attention to the other traditional cardiac risk factors and identify all the ones you have.

- *Smoking*
- *High blood pressure:* Greater than 140/90 mm Hg or >135/85 mm Hg if a diabetic (count high blood pressure as a risk factor if you are taking any blood pressure medications, even if your blood pressure is controlled).
- *Family history of coronary heart disease:* Male relative less than age 55 years or female relative less than 65 years.
- *Age:* Men 45 years old and above; women 55 years old and above.
- *Obesity:* BMI >30 or waist size in men >40 in. or women >35 in.

Identify markers of high risk

Step 3: There are some factors that move you right to the head of the heart disease risk line, although this is one line you would rather be in the back of (or not in line at all). All of these factors are associated with the highest risk for developing coronary artery disease and its complications. If you have any of these factors, be on high alert for problems and take every measure you can to lower your risk.

- *Diabetes mellitus:* Type 1 or Type 2.
- *Metabolic syndrome:* If you have at least three of the following five factors you have the metabolic syndrome.

Risk Factor	Defining Level
Abdominal obesity	Waist circumference
Men	>40 in.
Women	>35 in.
Triglycerides	>150 mg/dL
HDL cholesterol	
Men	<40 mg/dL
Women	<50 mg/dL
Blood pressure	>130/>85 mm Hg
Fasting blood glucose	>110 mg/dL

- *Carotid artery disease:* Blockage in carotid arteries or prior stroke.

- *Peripheral vascular disease:* Blockage in leg arteries or symptoms of "claudications."

- *Abdominal aortic aneurysm:* An enlarged aorta (measured by CT scan or ultrasound).

- *Known history of coronary artery disease:* Prior myocardial infarction, angioplasty or stent, coronary artery bypass surgery, or documented disease by abnormal stress test or angiography.

Consider digging a little deeper

Step 4: If you really want to know your cardiac risk, you have to be aggressive and dig a little deeper than just checking your cholesterol levels. That's where the emerging cardiac risk factors and some of the new imaging and diagnostic tests come into play.

Here is a review of some of the more commonly available and important ways to help evaluate your cardiac risk. I encourage you to always use these tests as an adjunct to the traditional cardiac risk factors.

Test	Defining Result
C-reactive protein	<1 mg/L = low risk
	1–3 mg/L = moderate risk
	>3 mg/L = high risk
Lipoprotein (a)	>30 mg/dL = higher risk

continued

Test	Defining Result
Homocysteine	5–15 umol/L = normal
	>15 umol/L = higher risk
Heart scan (EBCT)	0 = extremely low risk
	1–10 = very low risk
	11–100 = intermediate risk
	101–400 = high risk
	>400 = very high risk
Carotid IMT	Abnormal thickening and plaque detection
BART	Abnormal arterial response to stress

Determine your risk

Step 5: Now let's put it all together. This is the easy part—gathering all the data above is what is going to take some effort and time on your part. Simply put, the more cardiac risk factors you identify, the higher your risk for coronary artery disease and its complications. I break down your risk level into three categories: *highest*, *higher*, and *lower risk*.

Highest Risk: Red Flag Danger Zone

You are at the highest risk of developing coronary artery disease or developing the complications of coronary artery disease (heart attack, heart surgeries, cardiac death) if you have any of the high-risk markers:

- Diabetes mellitus
- Metabolic syndrome
- Carotid artery disease
- Peripheral vascular disease
- Abdominal aortic aneurysm
- Known history of coronary artery disease

You are also at the highest risk if you have *any* of these factors:

- Three or more cardiac risk factors (traditional and/or emerging)
- Coronary artery calcium score greater than 100
- Markedly elevated C-reactive protein (on multiple checks)

Higher Risk: Take Aggressive Measures

You are at least moderate risk, or "higher" risk for coronary artery disease and its complications, if you have any of these factors:

- Two cardiac risk factors (traditional and/or emerging)
- Moderately elevated C-reactive protein (on multiple checks)
- Coronary artery calcium score greater than 10

Lower Risk: Keep Up the Good Work!

You are at low risk for developing coronary artery disease at its complications if you can claim to have

- Zero or one cardiac risk factor (as long as it's not diabetes—see highest risk)

There are also some test results that can help put you in the lower-risk category. No matter what your test results, however, always factor in your total number of cardiac risk factors to gauge your overall cardiac risk.

- A coronary artery calcium score <10
- Normal C-reactive protein levels

Cardiac Risk Assessment Based on the Framingham Heart Study

This risk calculator is a common way to help assess your overall risk for developing angina, heart attack, or sudden cardiac death over the course of ten years. Separate score sheets are used for men and women. I have provided the score sheets based on LDL cholesterol, which I prefer over the ones based on total cholesterol (which are available at www.nhlbi.nih.gov).

Symbol	Risk
*	Very Low
**	Low
***	Moderate
****	High
*****	Very High

The authors of this risk algorithm urge you to be aware of a few caveats:

- These risk score sheets are for persons without known heart disease.
- The Framingham Heart Study population is almost all Caucasian; therefore this algorithm may not fit other populations as well.
- The Framingham risk score estimates the risk of developing coronary heart disease (CHD) within a ten-year period. The long-term risk or lifetime risk of developing CHD is one in two for men and one in three for women.
- The presence of any CHD risk factor requires appropriate attention because a single risk factor may confer a high risk for CHD in the long run (even if your score here does not appear to be high).
- The score derived from this algorithm should not be used as a substitute for an evaluation by your doctor.

Framingham Risk Algorithm for Men

Step 1: What is your age?

Age (Years)	Points
30–34	–1
35–39	0
40–44	1
45–49	2
50–54	3
55–59	4
60–64	5
65–69	6
70–74	7

Step 2: What is your bad (LDL) cholesterol?

LDL Cholesterol (mg/dL)	Points
<100*	−3
100–129**	0
130–159***	0
160–189****	1
>190*****	2

Step 3: What is your good (HDL) cholesterol?

HDL Cholesterol (mg/dL)	Points
<35*****	2
35–44****	1
45–49***	0
50–59**	0
≥60*	−1

Step 4: What is your blood pressure?

Blood Pressure

Systolic (mm Hg)	Diastolic (mm Hg)				
	<80	80–84	85–89	90–99	>100
<120	0 points*	0**	1***	2****	3*****
120–129	0**	0 points**	1***	2****	3*****
130–139	1***	1***	1 point***	2****	3*****
140–159	2****	2****	2****	2 points****	3*****
≥160	3*****	3*****	3*****	3*****	3 points*****

Step 5: Do you have diabetes?

Diabetes	Points
No	0**
Yes	2*****

Step 6: Do you smoke?

Smoker	Points
No	0**
Yes	2*****

Step 7: Add up your points from steps 1 to 6.

Steps	Points
Age	_____
LDL cholesterol	_____
HDL cholesterol	_____
Blood pressure	_____
Diabetes	_____
Smoker	_____
Points total	_____

Step 8: Based on your points, determine your ten-year risk of developing coronary heart disease.

Coronary Heart Disease Risk

Points Total	Ten-Year CHD Risk
≤−3	1%
−2	2%
−1	2%
0	3%
1	4%
2	4%
3	6%
4	7%
5	9%
6	11%

Points Total	Ten-Year CHD Risk
7	14%
8	18%
9	22%
10	27%
11	33%
12	40%
13	47%
≥14	≥55%

Step 9: Compare your calculated risk to that of a healthy man your age without any cardiac risk factors; this gives your relative risk of developing CHD (see example score sheet, p. 181).

Comparative Risk

Age (Years)	Low Ten-Year CHD Risk
30–34	2%
35–39	3%
40–44	4%
45–49	4%
50–54	6%
55–59	7%
60–64	9%
65–69	11%
70–74	14%

Framingham Risk Algorithm for Women

Step 1: What is your age?

Age (Years)	Points
30–34	–9
35–39	–4
40–44	0
45–49	3
50–54	6
55–59	7
60–64	8
65–69	8
70–74	8

Step 2: What is your bad (LDL) cholesterol?

LDL Cholesterol (mg/dL)	Points
<100	–2*
100–129	0**
130–159	0***
160–189	2****
>190	2*****

Step 3: What is your good (HDL) cholesterol?

HDL Cholesterol (mg/dL)	Points
<35*****	5*****
35–44****	2****
45–49***	1***
50–59**	0**
≥60*	–2*

Step 4: What is your blood pressure?

Blood Pressure

Systolic (mmHg)	Diastolic (mm/Hg)				
	<80	80–84	85–89	90–99	>100
<120	–3 points*	0**	0***	2****	3*****
120–129	0**	0 points**	0***	2****	3*****
130–139	0***	0***	0 points***	2****	3*****
140–159	2****	2****	2****	2 points****	3*****
≥160	3*****	3*****	3*****	3*****	3 points*****

Step 5: Do you have diabetes?

Diabetes	Points
No	0**
Yes	4*****

Step 6: Do you smoke?

Smoker	Points
No	0**
Yes	2*****

Step 7: Add up your points from steps 1 to 6.

Steps	Points
Age	_____
LDL cholesterol	_____
HDL cholesterol	_____
Blood pressure	_____
Diabetes	_____
Smoker	_____
Points total	_____

Step 8: Based on your points, determine your ten-year risk of developing coronary heart disease.

Coronary Heart Disease Risk

Points Total	Ten-Year CHD Risk
≤−2	1%
−1	2%
0	2%
1	2%
2	3%
3	3%
4	4%
5	5%
6	6%
7	7%
8	8%
9	9%
10	11%
11	13%
12	15%
13	17%
14	20%
15	24%
16	27%
≥17	>32%

Step 9: Compare your calculated risk to that of a healthy women your age without any cardiac risk factors; this gives your relative risk of developing CHD (see example score sheet, p. 181).

Comparative Risk

Age (Years)	Low Ten-Year CHD Risk
30–34	<1%
35–39	<1%
40–44	2%

Age (Years)	Low Ten-Year CHD Risk
45–49	3%
50–54	5%
55–59	7%
60–64	8%
65–69	8%
70–74	8%

Sample Framingham CHD Risk Score Sheet

Man
Age: 57
LDL cholesterol: 165 mg/dL
HDL cholesterol: 34 mg/dL
Blood pressure: 147/85 mm Hg
Diabetes: No
Smoker: Yes

Step	Factor	Points
1	Age: 57	4
2	LDL cholesterol: 165 mg/dL	1
3	HDL cholesterol = 34	2
4	Blood pressure: 147/85	2
5	Diabetes: No	0
6	Smoker: Yes	2
7	Points total	11
8	Estimate ten-year CHD risk	33%
9	Look at risk of someone your age without major CHD risk factors	7%
10	Calculate your relative risk of developing CHD (step 8 divided by step 9)	33/7 = 4.7

This man is almost 5 times (4.7) more likely to develop a heart attack, angina, or sudden cardiac death than someone his age without these cardiac risk factors.

No matter what risk category you fall in, there is always room for improvement when trying to lead a heart-healthy lifestyle. Read on to the final phase of my program, Step Five, to find out how you can get yourself into, or keep yourself in, the lower-risk category to prevent coronary artery disease and heart attacks.

Live the Heart Smart Life: A Cardiologist's Practical and Proven Approach

N ow that you've got the information you need, it's time to make your move. It's time to *take action*! Preventing heart disease is not only possible, but it's also practically guaranteed if you follow the Heart Smart program.

Step Five of the program introduces you to a no-nonsense, straightforward, proven, and effective strategy to prevent, treat, and reverse coronary heart disease. This Heart Smart strategy puts you in control of your heart health. It encourages you to make exercise and fitness a central part of your life. It encourages you to choose foods that are good for your heart and don't cause obesity. As you'll see, the Heart Smart way of life involves more than just avoiding Big Macs. Living Heart Smart encompasses all aspects of your life.

As you've seen throughout this book, there are no shortcuts to heart disease prevention. But by following the approach detailed in this section, you can start to live—and continue living—a heart-healthy lifestyle. So don't wait for your heart to break down before you start taking care of it. Take responsibility for your heart health now and start living the Heart Smart life.

Chapter 11

Kick Off Your Heart Smart Program

101 Things You Can Do Now to Prevent a Heart Attack

People always ask me, "Is there anything I can do to get my heart into shape and lower my risk for a heart attack?"

My answer is always the same, "Yes, there are a ton of things you can do." And I made a list of specific steps to follow. Trust me, advice such as "Get more exercise" or "Eat less fat" just isn't going to cut it. You need to follow a specific list of *action items* to kick off your Heart Smart Program effectively. These action items are things you can do every day as part of your normal routine—at the grocery store, at work, at the gym, on vacation, and in the kitchen.

Don't wait any longer. Start reading, and start making the right decisions that will help you lose weight, feel stronger, look better, and live longer.

The Heart Smart 101

The Heart Smart Fundamentals

Use common sense; it will take you farther than you think.

Keep your Heart Smart plan simple, and stick to it.

Make Heart Smart decisions every day.

Never think of "going on a diet"; just start eating heart-healthy, nutritious food.

Avoid gimmicks, fads, and Internet scams.

185

Don't wait for a magic shortcut before you make a change; there are no shortcuts.

Be aggressive; find out your cardiac risk and fight to keep it low.

Seek out a physician who *knows and cares about* heart disease prevention.

Manage Your Traditional Cardiac Risks

Maintain a normal blood pressure of 120/80 mm Hg.

Make sure your fasting blood sugar level is less than 100 mg/dL.

Keep your triglycerides at less than 150 mg/dL.

Keep your LDL cholesterol at less than 100 mg/dL.

Keep your HDL cholesterol as high as you can get it (at least greater than 40 mg/dL).

Measure your waist and learn your body mass index (BMI). Maintain an ideal weight.

Learn your family's heart history.

Have a *no tolerance* policy for smoking and tobacco use.

Check Out Your Emerging Risk Factors

Check your CRP level to find out if you are at risk for a heart attack.

Check your LDL cholesterol pattern to see if it's "small and dangerous."

Find out how good your good cholesterol is by checking your HDL2b level.

Look out for the heart attack spark Lp(a).

Check to see if an elevated homocysteine level could be the cause of your early heart attack.

Find Out the Health of Your Arteries

Check the health of your arterial endothelium by doing a brachial artery reactivity test.

Look for early cholesterol buildup in your carotid arteries to gauge how your heart is doing (take the carotid arteries intima-media thickness test).

Make sure you know your coronary artery calcium score (measured during a heart scan or EBCT); it could save your life.

Manage Your Stress

As they say, don't sweat the small stuff.

Put some fun back into your life.

Remember what's important in life; your health is at the top of the list.

Get tired of being tired; get plenty of sleep.

Find something to laugh about every day.

Get a stress-free pet.

Exercise for Life

Engage in moderate-intensity exercise for forty-five to sixty minutes a day, five or more days a week.

Start with light activity and work your way up to more intense exercise.

Make exercise a part of your daily routine; schedule it in your day planner.

Set realistic goals and write them down.

Learn how to stretch before and after workouts to avoid injury.

Review and update your motivation to exercise.

Diversify your exercise routine to keep it interesting.

Choose activities that fit your abilities and interests.

Splurge on quality, comfortable gear up front.

Buy an iPod or other portable music player so you enjoy yourself while you exercise.

Don't let bad weather be an excuse; expect the worst and plan for it.

Expect good days and bad days; stay positive!

Avoid and Limit the Bad Fats

Limit your saturated-fat intake to less than 7 percent of your daily calories.

Avoid at all costs foods containing trans, hydrogenated, or partially hydrogenated fats.

Avoid or at least limit commercially fried or baked goods such as French fries, doughnuts, cookies, and crackers.

Attack your snack habits: replace potato chips and cookies with heart-healthy munchies.

Embrace and Increase the Good Fats

Make sure monounsaturated and polyunsaturated fats make up 20 to 25 percent of your daily calories.

Eat "oily" fish, such as salmon, tuna, mackerel, or herring, at least twice a week.

Consider adding omega-3 fatty acid supplements (1 gram a day) to your daily intake.

Eat a handful of peanuts, walnuts, almonds, or other nuts every day.

Use canola, olive, peanut, and safflower oil instead of hydrogenated vegetable oil.

Try avocados as a great heart-healthy snack.

Make Heart Smart Decisions When Shopping

Learn how to read and understand food labels.

Always choose lean meats: round steak, sirloin tip, extra-lean ground beef, pork tenderloin, center-cut loin chops, lamb loin chops.

Choose chicken breasts or drumsticks instead of wings and thighs.

Buy foods that are fat-free or low-fat, cholesterol-free, or low-cholesterol.

Stick with low-salt, salt-free, or no-salt-added products.

Avoid potato chips, tortilla chips, and snack crackers that are fried.

Go with 1 percent or fat-free milk (an eight-ounce glass of 2 percent milk has the equivalent of one whole tablespoon of butter in it).

Bypass the ice cream and frozen desserts.

Look for low-saturated-fat, whole-grain breakfast cereals.

Learn How to Eat Heart Healthy When You're Eating Out or Traveling

Limit eating out to no more than once a week.

Avoid liquid calories; most big-brand soda products contain ten to twelve teaspoons of sugar per twelve-ounce drink.

Order one meal and split it with someone.

Save ten grams of fat and ninety calories by putting nonfat whipped cream on your Starbucks mocha rather than using whipped cream or whole milk.

Use the doggie bag early and often.

Stay away from "all you can eat" buffets.

Resist the urge to supersize any food item.

If you get a burger, eat it without mayo, cheese, fries, or a shake.

Stick to grilled chicken, grilled fish, salads, veggies, and fruit.

Avoid the appetizers; very few are heart-healthy.

Learn How to Cook Heart Smart

Eliminate the skin on poultry; stick with skinless white meat.

Limit rich sauces and creams; skim the fat off pan drippings; for cream sauces, use skim milk and soft tub or liquid margarine.

Prepare foods by steaming, broiling, baking, or grilling rather than frying.

Use margarine as a substitute for butter.

Use soy or tofu as a protein substitute.

Experiment with herbs and spices while limiting salt and butter.

Buy a Heart Smart cooking guide.

Learn about and follow the Mediterranean Diet.

Cut way back on cheese, please: a typical serving contains as much saturated fat as about three or four pats of butter.

Keep Your Diet in Good Balance

Limit the simple sugars and carbohydrates to about 50 percent of your daily calories.

Shop regularly for fresh fruit.

Make whole grains a healthy addition to your diet routine.

Eat whole wheat pasta, brown rice, and whole-grain flours, cereals, and breads.

Limit the sweets and desserts to once a week.

Drink alcohol in moderation only (and know what moderation means).

Redefine Your Portions

Slowly dial back on your portion sizes.

Never have seconds.

Curb your hunger pains by eating more filling proteins and good fats.

Remember that a portion of meat is about the size of a deck of cards—not a Frisbee.

Eat Heart Smart Superfoods

Try using two or three helpings of a stanol/sterol spread in place of butter a day.

Look to soy protein to lower your cholesterol: try edamame (Japanese soybeans), soymilk, tofu, and soybean burgers.

Use garlic to flavor a few meals a week.

Get your vitamin E through a balanced diet and foods containing antioxidants (vegetables and whole grains), not with supplements.

Add some foods that are rich in fiber: apples, figs, beets, Brussels sprouts, sweet potatoes, baked beans, chickpeas, pinto beans, brown rice, bran flakes, oatmeal, and nuts.

Take Advantage of Heart Smart Drugs

Consider taking a coated baby aspirin a day to prevent heart attacks and strokes.

Remember that cholesterol-lowering drugs, such as the statins, can reduce your risk of a heart attack by a third or more.

Don't be afraid of niacin; it's the best drug for bringing up your good HDL cholesterol and for lowering your lipoprotein(a) level.

Be patient with blood pressure medication; it may take a few tries before you find one that works well.

Ask your doctor about combination drugs for blood pressure and cholesterol to simplify your life.

I hope this list encourages you to take action! Remember, decisions you make throughout the day affect your heart and your health. Try to make Heart Smart decisions!

Chapter 12

Exercise

A Priority for Heart Health

Imagine a treatment that could lower your risk of cardiovascular disease and diabetes, lower your blood pressure, lower your cholesterol, help you lose weight, improve your bone strength, make you happier, and help improve the way you look. Now imagine that this treatment was all-natural, had no major side effects, was available anytime, didn't require a prescription, and was completely free.

Sound too good to be true? It's not. The treatment, of course, is exercise, and beginning an exercise regimen is one of the best things you can do to start preventing heart disease.

Unfortunately, exercise is not a priority in most of our lives. We are a nation of active sports *fans* rather than active sports *participants*. The sedentary American lifestyle is literally killing us. Our children are headed for unheard-of levels of obesity and eventually coronary heart disease because they're growing up in a world of high-tech gadgets, video games, and 160-channel television sets, with little time for or interest in exercise.

Let's face it: kids learn by example, and the lessons they are learning from adults is that a new TiVo is more important than a gym membership, that exercise takes a backseat to work, and that fast food is better than healthy food. But to prevent coronary heart disease, as well as to feel

---

Heart Smart Fact

The average American now watches almost four hours of television a day, which amounts to *sixty days* of idle time spent in front of the television per year.

191

better and enjoy a new and improved self-image, you need to understand the importance of exercise—and make it a priority. *It's every bit as powerful and effective—and as important—as any medicine you will ever take.*

What Is Exercise and How Much Do You Need?

Exercise is any physical activity or bodily movement that expends energy or calories. While all exercise is beneficial, and everyone will have a different fitness goal, the American Heart Association and the Centers for Disease Control recommend that you "Engage in moderate-intensity physical activities for at least forty-five to sixty minutes a day on five or more days per week." This rigorous type of activity will burn 3.5 to 7 calories per minute (kcal/min) and increase both your heart rate and your breathing rate; you'll be able to tell that your heart is getting a workout.

Moderate-intensity activities are suggested because they provide the most "bang for your buck." Light-intensity exercises are beneficial, but you need to spend more time doing them (at least an hour a day) to get the same health benefits as moderate-intensity activities (forty-five to sixty minutes a day). Vigorous activities are okay, too, but they increase your risk of injury while not providing you with additional health benefits.

Moderate-intensity activities
- Playing volleyball
- Walking two miles
- Shooting baskets
- Bicycling five miles
- Dancing
- Water aerobics
- Walking eighteen holes of golf
- Running 1½ miles
- Gardening
- Pushing a stroller
- Stair-walking

The Three Exercise Variables

Your exercise prescription includes three variables: length of time, frequency, and intensity. When starting any kind of exercise program, be sure to keep all three in mind. The length of time you exercise should be at least forty-five to sixty minutes, the number of times you exercise should be at least five days a week, and your exercise intensity level should be at least moderate, to take advantage of exercise's health benefits.

What Are the Benefits of Exercise?

Regular moderate-intensity exercise significantly cuts your risk for developing coronary heart disease and slashes your risk of dying from it by *a half*. But not only that; it also benefits every controllable cardiac risk factor. It prevents or reverses high blood pressure, high LDL cholesterol, low HDL cholesterol, diabetes, the metabolic syndrome, obesity, and stress—and it benefits you even if you already have heart disease.

Exercise Lowers High Blood Pressure

A variety of different exercises have now been proven to lower blood pressure. Circuit weight training, resistance training, and aerobic training all have been shown to reduce systolic blood pressure by as much as 12 mm Hg and to reduce diastolic blood pressure by as much as 8 mm Hg.

Exercise seems to "readjust" your body's blood pressure gauge downward and lower your resting heart rate. Exercise's positive effects on blood pressure can be seen in as few as four to five weeks.

Heart Smart Exercise Tip

Exercise is the *single most effective* way for you to lower your risk of heart attacks, high cholesterol, high blood pressure, diabetes, and obesity.

Exercise Lowers Bad Cholesterol and Raises Good Cholesterol

Exercise has a beneficial effect on all the major lipids. Regular moderate-intensity exercise lowers total cholesterol by up to 13 percent, raises HDL cholesterol levels 2 to 4 percent (remember, for every 1 percent increase in HDL, your risk of coronary heart disease will be lowered by 2 percent), and lowers LDL cholesterol by up to 15 percent. Your triglycerides are especially sensitive to the effects of exercise and can be lowered by 20 percent or more.

Exercise Prevents Diabetes

Exercise has a number of benefits that help prevent diabetes if you don't have it and limits the effects of the disease if you do have it. If you do have diabetes, exercise will lower your blood glucose levels and tissue energy stores, improve insulin sensitivity, and promote weight loss. It is particularly valuable if you have Type 2 diabetes because it lowers blood pressure, lowers triglyceride levels, raises HDL levels, and helps you lose weight, all key to managing the disease.

One of the biggest problems living with Type 2 diabetes, the metabolic syndrome, and prediabetes is insulin resistance. If you have insulin resistance, you have plenty of insulin in your bloodstream, but your cells' insulin receptors are resistant to its effects. Exercise can actually reverse resistance to insulin. It not only improves your cells' ability to pick up insulin, it also increases the number of healthy insulin receptors.

If you are a diabetic and want to start an exercise program, make sure you check with your doctor first to see if your medications need to be adjusted and if you need to take a stress test before beginning.

Exercise Washes Away Stress

How you handle the stress of the everyday rat race significantly impacts your risk for heart attacks and cardiovascular disease. Stress, anger, and anxiety can contribute to an unhealthy lifestyle and cardiovascular disease.

No other treatment or prescription drug does more to help relieve stress and anger than exercise. It does so in several different ways: by providing an outlet for anger, by helping you relax strained muscles through repetitive tense-and-release motions, and by providing social support and the human connection if you exercise with a group or participate in a team sport. If you enjoy exercising on your own, it gives you time for solitude and introspection.

Exercise's Big Plus

In addition to improving your heart health and providing critical stress relief, exercise also enables you to take some most likely much-needed personal time. Putting the job on hold or taking a break from the kids' endless needs to go running or bicycling can do wonders to improve your outlook.

Exercise also can simply make you feel better. Research suggests that exercise may trigger the release of endorphins, special hormones that are thought to produce the "high" that some people feel with activity. Endorphins act like morphine, providing pain relief and inducing a feeling of euphoria.

Because it can prevent disease, relieve stress, and give you a new sense of self-esteem and confidence, exercise is a critical component of the Heart Smart way of living.

How to Make Exercise a Regular Part of Your Life

If you're chomping at the bit to get your new exercise program under way, that's great—I applaud you. But before you jump in, take a few minutes to think about the following. Starting off on the right foot will help ensure that exercise becomes an important, exciting, and long-term part of your life.

Review Your Motivation

There are a lot of great motivating factors to help you start and stay on a regular exercise program. If you need more motivation than "My doctor told me to do it," which may not be enough to keep you exercising for the long haul, consider exercising to lose weight, to look and feel better, to meet new friends, to become more social, to become competitive, or to have a great source of stress relief.

Whatever your motivation, use it to help you keep exercising for all the years ahead.

Choose the Right Activities

Everyone has different physical skills, limitations, and restrictions. The key is to make exercise a personal choice that fits your lifestyle, personality, and abilities. Some people like the solitude of a long walk in the park or on the beach; others like the team effort and camaraderie that come with playing basketball or volleyball. Don't pick an activity just because your spouse or friends are involved in it; pick something you want to do and will enjoy and then *go for it.*

If you find that you chose the wrong activity, it's not the end of the world. Don't get frustrated and give up. Be sure to start your exercise plan with the expectation that you might need to pick a new activity, change where or when you exercise, or change your exercise goals. Don't let the wrong activity put you off exercise completely.

Diversify Your Exercise Plan

Your interest in exercise should stay strong if you stay involved in several different activities. Diversifying helped one of my patients go from doing no exercise to exercising five or six days a week.

Jason started his exercise program by doing the same routine at the same workout facility every other day, but he quickly became bored with it. I encouraged him to rotate among several different types of workouts, and he hasn't slowed down since.

Two days a week Jason works out at the gym with a combination of aerobic "cardio" exercises and light strength/resistance training. Two days a week he plays in a men's tennis league, and one to two days a week he rides his bike with his wife. If the weather is bad he rides a stationary bike or picks up a game of basketball. Not only do all of these workouts make Jason feel great, but they've also enabled him to develop a new social network and a new set of friends.

By diversifying your exercise routine you are more likely to stay involved with exercise for the long run, avoid seasonal and weather limitations, work different sets of muscle groups, and avoid becoming stagnant.

Avoid Beginner's Injury

One of the biggest mistakes I see people making as they begin an exercise regimen is trying to do too much too soon. You may be surprised at what a shock exercise is to your body if you haven't been active in a few months or years.

To avoid injuring yourself as you start, and to keep from having your motivation crushed, follow these four recommendations:

1. *Pick an easy, light form of exercise*. Your goal may be to windsurf, but spending a month or two getting your body ready for such strenuous activity will help you reach your goal in one piece.

2. *Try to stick with low-impact exercise*. Your bones, back, joints, and tendons will thank you for picking activities that limit stress on them.

3. *Start slowly*. You do not need to make up for the past three years of inactivity in the first week of your new exercise program. I advise my patients to start two or three exertion levels below where they think they should start and to work up slowly over weeks, not days.

4. *Each time you exercise, make sure to include adequate warm-up and cool-down times*. Spending just a few minutes warming up and stretching out will significantly reduce your chance of injury and get your body in a "ready state" for being active. Cooling down will also help to prevent injury and smooth the transition back to your preactivity state.

Set Goals

Goal-setting can improve all aspects of your life. From saving money to losing weight, setting and writing down goals—and sharing them with your friends or family—will give you a much better chance of success.

Exercise is no different. Setting goals for your activity will help you make and work at keeping a long-term commitment to a heart-healthy lifestyle.

Elizabeth had been exercising on and off for years. During the longer days of summer she had no problems exercising four or five times a week. In the winter, however, she just never could seem to find the time (or daylight) to keep up with her exercise regimen. Between holiday eating splurges and the drop-off in her exercise, Elizabeth always managed to gain eight to ten pounds each winter season.

Two years ago I helped Elizabeth set up and write down some goals to help get her motivated to stay healthy over the wintertime. Elizabeth's goals were to play in a volleyball league once a week, complete a fitness circuit at the gym twice a week, and to maintain her weight. Elizabeth not only met her goals by writing them down, she even exceeded them by actually losing a few pounds.

When you review your motivation for exercising, set goals to match—don't just start exercising randomly with no specific target. Whether your goal is to finish a five-K race, to walk eighteen holes of golf, to be able to walk to the top of the trail by your house, to lose fifteen pounds, or to get into that smaller dress or pair of pants, goals will help you stick with your exercise program. But if you don't reach your goals, try not to become frustrated. You may need to reevaluate them and adjust them if they are unrealistic.

Make Exercise a Habit

The people I know who exercise most consistently have made exercise a part of their daily routine. Instead of always trying to squeeze exercise into their busy schedule or rearrange things at the last minute to include it, it's on the calendar and takes place like clockwork. These people never even have to think about when they'll exercise; it's scheduled and it just happens.

Exercise needs to be both a priority and a habit in your life. To keep yourself from finding excuses, such as you have no time or you're too busy, make physical activities—your early-morning visit to the gym, a lunchtime walk, the weekly tennis match—part of your schedule and part of your routine.

Make Exercise Fun

Exercise provides serious health and wellness benefits, but it should also be fun, so be sure to choose a sport or an activity you really enjoy. Join a

---

Heart Smart Fact

Compared to being sedentary, exercise single-handedly cuts your risk of developing cardiovascular disease in half!

gym and make new friends, get some buddies together and form a hiking club, make exercise a family affair by involving your kids and spouse, rekindle that old competitive spirit and join a team. Whatever activity you pick, make exercise something you look forward to and have a great time doing. Put some fun back into your life with physical fitness.

Heart Rate Zones

Once you are comfortably back into exercising, you can start targeting specific heart rate zones based on your exercise goals. To check your heart rate you can either buy a heart rate monitor or take your pulse on your own.

Heart rate monitors are accurate and relatively inexpensive, depending on how many bells and whistles you want. The least expensive route, though, is to count your own heart rate by checking your pulse. To check your pulse, put your index finger on your neck (carotid artery) or the inside of your wrist (radial artery). The carotid artery pulse is on the side of your neck between the middle of your collarbone and your jawline. The radial artery pulse is found by turning your hand palm up and feeling for the pulse at the base of your thumb, way off to the side of the wrist.

When you feel the pulse, count the number of beats for 60 seconds to find out your resting heart rate. You can use a shortcut by counting your pulse for 6 seconds and then multiplying that number by 10; by counting it for 10 seconds and multiplying by 6; by counting for 15 seconds and multiplying by 4; or by counting for 30 seconds and multiplying by 2. All of these measurements will give you a fairly accurate heart rate.

When Bob, who is fifty, wanted to start a new fitness program to help him lose ten pounds and lower his cholesterol, he began by determining his maximum heart rate (MHR). The maximum heart rate is the level you should not exceed during exercise. To figure out your MHR, you simply subtract your age from 220. Bob's MHR is 220–50, or 170 beats per minute.

After Bob determined his MHR, he then needed to figure out the best zone to keep his heart rate in to reach his exercise and fitness goals. Since Bob hadn't exercised in a while, he needed to start out nice and easy, so he began his exercise program with the goal of keeping his heart rate in the *warm-up zone*.

The Warm-Up Zone

The warm-up zone keeps your heart rate at a level that is 50 to 60 percent of your MHR. For Bob that's 85 to 102 beats per minute ($220-50 = 170 \times .5 = 85; 220-50 = 170 \times .6 = 102$).

The warm-up zone is a good target for a five- to ten-minute warm-up or a great place to begin if you are just starting an exercise program.

The Heart Smart Fitness Zone

The Heart Smart fitness zone is 60 to 70 percent of your MHR. For Bob this means between 102 and 119 beats per minute. By keeping your heart rate in this zone you will see such positive results as weight loss, lower blood pressure, lower cholesterol, and improved fitness.

The Heart Smart fitness zone is the zone I encourage most of my older patients to aim for. It's considered moderate exertion for most older and out-of-shape people, yet it provides cardiovascular and health benefits with regular exercise.

The Aerobic Zone

If your heart is beating at 70 to 80 percent of your MHR, you're exercising in the aerobic zone. To exercise in this zone Bob needs to raise his heart rate to 119 to 136 beats per minute.

This zone not only improves your cardiovascular health but actually helps strengthen your heart. And since up to 85 percent of calories burned in this zone are from fat, it's also a great zone to work out in if you want to lose weight. *If you are younger, relatively healthy, training for competitive events, or desire maximum cardiovascular benefits from your exercise, this is the zone for you.*

The Anaerobic Zone

The anaerobic zone is centered on a heart rate that's 80 to 90 percent of your MHR. Bob will never need to target his heart rate for this zone, because endurance is not one of his goals. If his goals change and he does want to aim for greater endurance, though, his heart rate goal would need to be 136 to 153 beats per minute.

If your goal is to run or swim competitively, or to increase your endurance as much as possible, then the anaerobic zone should be your target zone.

The Maximum Zone

This zone requires you to exercise very intensely—you need to keep your heart rate at 90 to 100 percent of your MHR. Bob's maximum zone would have his heart pumping between 153 and 170 beats per minute, but again, this is not a zone he would target.

Most people, in fact, do not need to exercise in this zone. You certainly will burn calories if you do, but working out at this high level does not give you any added cardiovascular health benefits. If you do decide you want to target your maximum zone, make sure you check with your doctor to determine if you are ready to do so safely.

Get It in Gear: Start Filling Your Exercise Prescription

Just like medication, regular moderate-intensity exercise plays a central role in the quest to prevent or treat coronary heart disease. So think of it not as something I suggest that you do, but as a real prescriptive treatment that your doctor is telling you to take. The kind of physical activity you do is completely up to you—it doesn't have to be anything fancy, brisk walking is just fine—but you need to do it five or more days a week for no less than forty-five to sixty minutes a day.

Your Exercise Prescription

R_x: Moderate-intensity exercise

Dosage: Once or twice a day for at least forty-five minutes a day

Frequency: Five or more days a week

Refills: For life (a long and healthy life)

Tips and Tricks for Happily Staying the Course

Now that you are mentally ready to start an exercise program, be sure to take the following important steps to prepare yourself to stay the course for the long run.

Splurge on Some Gear

Before you start your exercise regimen, reward yourself for taking on the challenge and spend some money on good equipment. Having the right gear often makes the difference between success and failure. Worn or poorly fitting shoes or equipment can cause injury and make enjoying exercise next to impossible.

For outdoor exercise I recommend that you wear comfortable shoes, athletic socks, sun protection, and all-weather gear. I also tell my patients to invest in an iPod, portable radio, or the like. Jamming to some of your favorite tunes, listening to a book on tape, or rooting for your favorite team while you exercise can help keep you pumped up and moving.

Don't Let the Weather Be an Excuse Not to Exercise

It's too hot. It's too cold. It's too wet. It's too windy. You would think a lot of people have never heard of jackets, gloves, rain gear, or hats. If you prepare yourself well (see above), Mother Nature won't slow you down, and you'll still be able to exercise comfortably. Just assume when you start your program that weather will be an issue at times, and either make plans to exercise indoors or have good protective gear at the ready.

Stay Hydrated

Your body needs to be well hydrated both during exercise and between exercise sessions. Even if you don't sweat a lot, you still need to drink extra fluids when you exercise. I recommend taking a water break at least every twenty minutes and more frequently at high altitudes, in hot weather, or during vigorous workouts.

Stay Positive!

Like anything else, you'll have good days working out, but you'll also have some not so good days. When things are less than great, try not to become frustrated or give up. The fun and satisfaction will kick back in, or if they don't, just try some other activities until you find something that really gets you going. Stay positive, set a good example, and keep working at it. Remember how important exercise is for both you and your family.

Don't Neglect a Heart-Healthy Diet

Exercise goes a long way in reestablishing good health, and it's a central part of a heart-healthy lifestyle. But once you start exercising it doesn't mean you can neglect other parts of your life. You'll maximize the benefits of exercise and achieve significant weight loss by combining exercise with heart-healthy eating, which we cover in the next chapter.

Summing It Up

Exercise is the single most important component of living a Heart Smart lifestyle. Regular, moderate-intensity exercise, for forty-five to sixty minutes a day, five or more days a week, is proven to lower your blood pressure, lower your cholesterol, help you lose weight, relieve stress, and substantially lower your risk of a heart attack. Put a little fun back into your life—ask your doctor to write you a prescription for exercise today.

Chapter 13

What Can I Eat?

The Heart Smart *Approach to Nutrition,
Dieting, Heart-Healthy "Superfoods,"
and Supplements*

Everywhere you turn you are bombarded with unhealthy foods that are literally choking off the blood supply to your heart. To live a heart-healthy lifestyle, you need to rethink and change your dangerous eating habits *now*!

And not just for a few weeks. Healthful eating needs to become a way of life, not a short-term solution to a problem. (The word "diet" implies a short-term solution, and diet fads have now become a multimillion-dollar industry; at the end of this chapter I'll give you a cardiologist's take on some of those diets, including the Atkins Diet, the South Beach Diet, and the Mediterranean Diet.) To be Heart Smart you need to adopt permanent heart-healthy dietary habits rather than jump on a six-week "miracle cure" or another fad or gimmick.

The Heart Smart Dietary Plan

Changing your habits may sound daunting, but it's really not. By following my easy-to-use Heart Smart nutrition guide, you can begin to make heart-healthy changes today. And once you've developed good habits, there will be no looking back. A well-balanced, nutritious diet will make you look and feel like a new person.

The Heart Smart dietary plan has four components that will minimize your risk of coronary heart disease:

1. Know your good fats from your bad fats.

2. Work toward a more balanced diet.

3. Rein in the size of your portions.

4. Learn about "superfoods" that promote heart health.

By taking these steps you will be pleasantly surprised at how easy it is to regain control of your eating habits, your weight, and your life.

1. Know Your Good Fats from Your Bad Fats

The first step to eating a heart-healthy diet is to be an informed consumer—be smart about what you are putting in your mouth. You don't need to have the knowledge of a dietician, but you should have some basic understanding of nutritional information.

The single biggest dietary emergency facing America today is that we eat much too much fat! And not only do we eat too much *fat*, but we also eat too much of the *wrong kind of fat*.

In chapter 6 you learned a little about the good fats and the bad fats. The good ones *improve* your heart health and lower your risk of dying from cardiovascular disease; the bad fats increase your risk of obesity, high LDL cholesterol, high triglycerides, low HDL cholesterol, and heart attacks. A critical step in preventing and reversing heart disease is cutting back on eating bad fats and eating a moderate amount of good fats.

The Basic Facts on Fat

Your body requires some fat for normal cell function and structure. Fat is a great energy source, helps build cell membranes, helps carry fat-soluble vitamins (A, D, E, and K), and plays a central role in maintaining healthy skin and hair. Fat also can help you eat less because it helps fill you up more quickly. Diets high in carbohydrates cause wide fluctuations of blood sugar and insulin levels, which often make you feel hungry soon after you finish eating. Fat, on the other hand, doesn't affect blood sugar levels as much, allowing you to feel full sooner. This means you can eat less, yet still satisfy your hunger.

But fat intake, even the good kind of fat, still has to be limited. All fats are high in calories, so eating them in excess leads to weight gain and obesity. Fats contain nine calories per gram; proteins and carbohydrates contain only four calories per gram.

The Four Types of Fats

There are four types of dietary fat: *saturated*, *trans*, *monounsaturated*, and *polyunsaturated*. Saturated and trans fats are the bad fats; monounsaturated and polyunsaturated fats are the good fats. The recommended total daily intake of both good and bad fats is 25 to 30 percent of your total calories.

Dietary Fats

Type of Fat	Major Sources	Effect on Blood Cholesterol Levels
Saturated	Butter, whole milk, cheese, ice cream; red meat; coconut oil, palm oil	Raises LDL cholesterol
Trans fatty acids or trans fats	Vegetable shortening, partially hydrogenated vegetable oil; potato chips; most commercially baked goods (cookies, doughnuts, cakes, muffins); French fries	Raises LDL cholesterol
Monounsaturated	Canola oil, olive oil, olives, peanut oils; most nuts, including cashews, almonds, and peanuts; avocados	Lowers LDL cholesterol; raises HDL cholesterol
Polyunsaturated	Soybean, safflower, corn, flaxseed, and cottonseed oils; oily fish; walnuts	Lowers LDL cholesterol; raises HDL cholesterol

Choose Your Oils Wisely

Monounsaturated vegetable oils reign supreme when it comes to your heart. Researchers point to olive oil in Mediterranean diets and canola oil

---

Heart Smart Fat Warning!

All fats are high in calories, so even the good fats must be eaten in moderation.

in Asian diets as key reasons why these populations are relatively heart disease–free. Simply changing from the dangerous oils (palm, palm kernel, coconut, and all-vegetable oils), loaded with saturated and trans fats, to the mono- and polyunsaturated heart-healthy oils will make a huge difference in lowering your cardiac risk.

Fat Composition of Oils (by percentage)

Type of Oil	Monounsaturated	Polyunsaturated	Saturated
Canola	62	32	6
Olive	77	9	14
Peanut	49	33	18
Safflower	13	77	10
Soybean	24	61	15
Walnut	19	67	14
Coconut	6	2	92
Palm	38	10	52
Palm kernel	12	2	86

Federal Guidelines on Fat Consumption

As the primary culprits that cause coronary heart disease and obesity, trans and saturated fats should be only a very limited part of your diet. The latest federal nutritional guidelines, called the Dietary Guidelines for Americans 2005, make the following recommendations for fat intake:

- Keep total fat intake between 20 and 35 percent of total calories, with most fats coming from polyunsaturated and monounsaturated fatty acid sources such as fish, nuts, and vegetable oils.

- Consume less than 10 percent of calories from saturated fatty acids; keep cholesterol intake to less than 300 mg/day; keep trans fatty acid consumption as low as possible.

- Limit intake of fats and oils high in saturated and/or trans fatty acids, and choose products low in such fats and oils.

I agree with these recommendations, unless you already have coronary artery disease or are at moderate to high risk for the disease; then, in my opinion, the guidelines are too lenient. The greater your risk of heart disease, the more stringent you should be with limiting your bad fat intake. There are very good data that prove that extremely low-fat diets even help reverse coronary artery disease, though these kinds of diets are difficult to adhere to in the long term.

Limit Total Daily Fat Intake

If you're at higher risk for heart disease, I recommend that your total fat intake be no more than 20 percent of your total daily calories. I also recommend that you eliminate trans fats altogether, cut unsaturated fats to less than 5 percent of total daily calories, and cut your cholesterol intake to less than 200 mg/day.

Read on for more information about increasing your good fat intake while trimming down your bad intake as part of a well-rounded, balanced Heart Smart diet.

2. Work toward a More Balanced Diet

The average American diet is completely out of balance: it's heavily laden with saturated fats and carbohydrates, leaving little or no room for fruits, vegetables, and grains. Even the latest trendy diets aim to keep you out of balance—most of the commonly followed low-carbohydrate diets take you from one extreme (too many carbs and not enough protein) to the other extreme (no carbs and too much protein).

The Heart Smart diet and prevention plan encourages you to regain your diet balance. It emphasizes moderation and a balance among all the healthy food groups, which is the best nutritional plan for your heart, weight, and overall health.

It's time to get your balance back. Let's look closely at some important things you can do to put together and follow a *well-balanced* Heart Smart diet.

Eliminate Saturated and Trans Fats

There are a number of simple ways by which you can cut back on your intake of saturated and trans fats:

- Choose lean meats.
- Buy foods that are fat-free or low-fat.
- Avoid eating poultry skin.

- Limit rich sauces and creams.
- Prepare foods by steaming, broiling, baking, or grilling rather than frying.
- Use margarine as a substitute for butter.
- Avoid commercially fried or baked goods such as French fries, doughnuts, cookies, and crackers.
- Learn how to read labels.
- Avoid foods labeled "trans," "hydrogenated," or "partially hydrogenated."

Also look beyond animal products, which contain cholesterol, for sources of protein. Legumes (beans, peas, and lentils) are good protein sources that have less fat and no cholesterol. You can also expand your horizons by trying soy protein as a substitute for animal protein.

Substitute Good Fats for Bad Fats

Start by changing the oils you cook with. Use canola, olive, peanut, or safflower oil instead of partially hydrogenated vegetable oils.

Next, make some changes in your nightly dinner entrée. Instead of eating red meat, substitute an oily fish, such as halibut, salmon, mackerel, or herring, at least twice a week. On other days try baked or grilled skinless chicken breasts and plenty of fruits, vegetables, and grains.

Finally, attack the snacks. Turn to heart-healthy munchies such as avocados and nuts rather than potato chips and cookies.

Eat More Fruits and Vegetables

Fruits and vegetables are rich in fiber, good sources of vitamins and minerals, and low in calories. They also help protect your heart because they contain phytochemicals that help prevent cardiovascular disease. Substitute fruits or vegetables for fat-filled snacks and for carbohydrate-heavy side dishes such as rice and potatoes.

Add Some Whole Grains

Whole grains are grains that have not had their bran and germ removed by milling, so they are good sources of fiber. They're also an excellent source of important vitamins and minerals.

Make whole grains part of your daily diet by eating whole-wheat pasta, brown rice, and whole grain–rich flours, cereals, and breads.

Limit Sweets and Salts

Our taste buds are being assaulted by too many extremely salty and extremely sweet foods. Most of us eat two to three times more salt on a daily basis than the recommended intake of 2.3 grams a day, and too much salt will contribute to high blood pressure. Sweets are high in calories and usually come wrapped in trans or saturated fats (cookies, cakes, etc.). Dietary sweets contribute to obesity, diabetes, and other cardiovascular risk factors.

To consume less salt, avoid canned foods such as soups, which are high in salt content. Eat more fresh foods and fewer salt-rich processed foods. Limit salt during cooking by sprinkling on herbs and spices for extra flavor instead of pouring on the salt, and finally, keep the saltshaker off the dining table. When your sweet tooth gets demanding, try a perfect piece of fruit or a fruit sorbet.

Drink Alcohol in Moderation

If you choose to drink alcohol, make sure you drink in moderation; the majority of people drink more alcohol than is considered to be heart-healthy. You'll receive the benefits of alcohol if you limit your consumption to four to five ounces of wine, twelve ounces of beer, or one to two ounces of eighty-proof whiskey a day.

3. Rein In the Size of Your Portions

Many of us have lost our common sense when it comes to food. We have a never-ending supply of every food under the sun, yet we eat each meal as though it might be made of the last morsels on Earth. Food portions have nearly doubled in the past fifteen years, and American restaurants serve portions that are up to 75 percent larger than their European counterparts. A recent study revealed that candy bars sold in the United States were 41 percent larger than the same product in Paris, soft drinks were 52 percent larger, and cartons of yogurt were a monstrous 82 percent larger.

This out-of-control portion size is a major contributing factor to cardiovascular disease and many of its risk factors, including obesity.

To eat a heart-healthy diet, you need to rein in your portion sizes. To do that, you need to begin by eating more slowly. Our on-the-go lifestyle has spilled over into our eating, and many of us now scarf food down so fast that our stomachs don't have time to tell our brains that we're full. When you're halfway done with your meal, take a five-minute break. After five minutes you may find that you're really not that hungry anymore.

A second thing you can do is cut your portions in half. You'll still be able to eat many of the foods you enjoy, but you won't get all the bad side effects of overdoing it. If you're at a restaurant, ask for a doggie bag early on. Put at least half your meal in the bag—restaurants often serve portions that are really big enough for two or three meals—and take it home to eat on another day.

Finally, try to avoid eating out as much as possible. It will be well worth the extra time it takes to pack a heart-healthy lunch rather than eat fast food every day. If you do need to eat in restaurants at times, be sure to avoid "all you can eat" buffets and supersize portions of anything.

If you slowly dial back your portion sizes, you will find that you don't need as much food to satisfy your hunger.

How Much Is a Single Serving?

Despite the ridiculously large portions we're served in restaurants, you may be shocked to find out that one serving of meat is only three to four ounces, roughly the size of a deck of cards. But rather than cut your portions to any particular size, I encourage you to simply cut them back slowly over the next six months. You will be pleasantly surprised at how easy it is to do.

---

4. Learn about "Superfoods" That Promote Heart Health

While you need to know which foods to avoid because they promote coronary heart disease, it's also important to know about the foods that help lower cholesterol and can even prevent heart attacks.

What are those foods? Fish, nuts, soy, garlic, and moderate amounts of alcohol may substantially lower your risk of cardiovascular disease.

Heart Smart Superfoods and Supplements

It's four o'clock on a Thursday afternoon and I finally get down to my last patient. I see that it's a young man of thirty-eight who wants some information about his cardiac risk. Great; I figure it should take me thirty minutes or so to tell him about cardiac risk factors and answer all his questions.

An hour and twenty minutes later and I was still trying to plow through Christian's extensive list of questions. "Are there foods that can lower my cholesterol or lower my risk of heart attack?" "How much fish do I really have to eat?"

"Is red wine or white wine better for my heart? What about beer?" "Vitamin E is good for the heart, isn't it?" "Larry King says I should take garlic for my heart. Is that true?" These are just a sampling of the questions Christian wanted me to answer to help separate the hype from the truth.

Since that day, I have kept an updated running list of heart-healthy foods and supplements at the ready. As you read in the previous chapter, eating foods that are low in saturated fat and cholesterol is a crucial piece of a heart-healthy diet. In addition, there are a number of specific foods that have been shown to help lower your risk of coronary heart disease and heart attacks. Finally, there are vitamins and supplements you can take to pump up your heart health even more. Read on to learn more about these special dietary additions and how to tell fact from fiction when it comes to their health effects.

Proven Heart Smart Foods and Supplements

- Omega-3 fatty acids
- Nuts
- Sterols and stanols
- Soy
- Alcohol in moderation
- Garlic
- Fiber

Omega-3 Fatty Acids: Eating Them Can Reduce Your Risk of Dying

Eskimos are Heart Smart! More than thirty years ago, researchers found that most Eskimos seemed immune to the damaging cardiovascular effects of eating a high-fat diet. They were eating a lot of fat, but it was the right kind of fat—so they were not dying from heart disease.

Their secret was that they were eating fats found in the oil of fish they were eating. These good kinds of fat are called omega-3 fatty acids.

How Do Omega-3 Fatty Acids Work?

Many doctors and most of my patients believe that the benefits omega-3 fatty acids provide are due to the acids' effects on cholesterol. Many doctors and most of my patients are wrong.

The omega-3 fatty acids also have other effects to help protect your heart: they *thin the blood by inhibiting platelet function, stabilize cholesterol plaque through some anti-inflammatory mechanisms, improve endothelial function, and lower blood pressure.* The exact mechanisms through which omega-3 fatty acids produce these benefits, however, is a matter of ongoing research and debate.

Omega-3 Oil (EPA and DHA) in Fish and Seafood

There are three types of omega-3 fatty acids. The first two, found primarily in oily fish such as salmon, are known as "long chain" omega-3 fatty acids. One is eicosapentaenoic acid (let's just call that EPA) and the other is decosahexaenoic acid (DHA). The third type of omega-3 fatty acid is called alphalinolenic acid (ALA); it's found in certain plant oils but not in fish.

EPA and DHA are polyunsaturated fats—good types of fat. They're both found almost exclusively in seafood, and their quantity varies depending on the type of fish. The types of fish that contain the highest levels of omega-3 fatty acids—that is, the most oily fish—are the most heart-healthy. These include tuna, sardines, salmon, mackerel, and herring.

The following table lists some of the most common types of seafood, their omega-3 oil content, and the number of ounces you need to eat to take in one gram of omega-3 fatty acids each day—the recommended dose if you have heart disease.

Type of Fish	Grams of Omega-3 Oil per 3-Oz. Serving	No. of Oz. per Day to Equal 1 Gram EPA/DHA
Tuna: light canned	0.26	12
Tuna: white canned	0.73	4
Tuna: fresh	0.24–1.28	2.5–12
Sardines	0.98–1.70	2–3
Salmon: pink	1.05	3
Salmon: Atlantic farmed	1.09–1.83	1.5–2.5
Mackerel	0.34–1.57	2–8.5
Herring: Pacific	1.81	1.5
Oyster: Pacific	1.17	2.5
Lobster	0.07–0.41	7.5–42.5
Crab: Alaskan king	0.35	8.5

Type of Fish	Grams of Omega-3 Oil per 3-Oz. Serving	No. of Oz. per Day to Equal 1 Gram EPA/DHA
Trout: farmed	0.98	3
Flounder/sole	0.42	7
Shrimp	0.27	11

Based on U.S. Department of Agriculture Nutrient Data Laboratory at www.nalusda.gov/fnic/foodcomp/.

Eating fish saves lives. Both very large and much smaller clinical trials around the world have pointed out this fact over and over. Substituting any polyunsaturated fat for a saturated or trans fat will lower your risk of coronary heart disease and heart attack, but consuming the polyunsaturated fat in omega-3 fatty acids is especially heart-healthy. Eating oily fish and other seafood can lower your risk of dying by up to 45 percent!

If you don't care for the taste of fish, don't despair. Heart-protective EPA and DHA are equally beneficial when taken as fish oil supplements (supplements are available in both 2:1 and 1:2 ratios; neither EPA nor DHA has been proven more beneficial than the other). I strongly encourage my patients with heart disease and those at high risk for heart disease to make EPA/DHA omega-3 fatty acids, in whatever form, part of their heart-healthy lifestyle.

How Much Fish Do You Need to Eat?

As I said earlier, the American Heart Association recommends that people with *known* heart disease eat one gram of EPA/DHA daily. But what if you're trying to keep from developing heart disease?

The Proven Benefits of Fish Oil Supplements

One of the largest studies that ever looked at the value of omega-3 fatty acid supplements was the GISSI-Prevention Study. In this trial, almost three thousand heart attack survivors were given 850-mg EPA/DHA capsules once a day for 3½ years. The results of the study were conclusive: death from any cause decreased by 20 percent and sudden cardiac death decreased by 45 percent when compared to heart attack survivors who did not take fish oil supplements.

If you have not been diagnosed with coronary heart disease and want to prevent sudden cardiac death and life-threatening heart rhythm problems, the recommendation is to eat oily fish at least twice a week or to take about 500 mg of an EPA/DHA supplement per day. However, I recommend a more aggressive approach for my patients who have multiple cardiac risk factors or who are at high risk for coronary heart disease. If you fall into one of those categories, you should take 1 gm of EPA/DHA a day.

The Fishy Side of Eating Fish

There are no major downsides to eating either of the recommended daily doses of omega-3 fatty acids. It may take some effort to learn to cook a variety of delicious heart-healthy fish dishes, but it will be well worth the effort.

There are, however, two concerns that some people have: about the mercury levels in fish and about the "fish burps" that sometimes result from taking EPA/DHA supplements.

Mercury   Mercury can "bioconcentrate" in fish at the top of the marine food chain, and consuming large amounts of it can potentially cause side effects. The FDA has issued an advisory for four species of fish in which mercury can bioconcentrate: king mackerel, shark, swordfish, and tile fish (or golden snapper).

If you are pregnant or breast-feeding, you should limit your intake of these four types of fish to no more than twice a week. For anyone who is not pregnant or breast-feeding, the risk of side effects or disease from mercury appears to be negligible but is a matter of ongoing debate.

Avoiding the "fish burp"   Fish oil capsules can be taken at any time, with or without meals. As the capsule dissolves in the stomach and releases its oil, some people experience a fishy burp. You can minimize this side effect by taking your capsules at bedtime, taking enteric-coated capsules, or taking capsules that you keep in the freezer.

ALA: The Plant Source for Omega-3 Fatty Acids

The plant source of omega-3 fatty acids is called ALA. Because your body doesn't make these essential acids, you need to eat them as part of your heart-healthy diet. ALA is found in

- Flaxseed oil (55 percent ALA by weight)
- Canola oil (11 percent ALA by weight)
- Soybeans

- Wheat germ
- Walnuts
- Pecans
- Pine nuts

Canola oil is probably the most likely source of ALA because it is readily found in salad and cooking oils, margarines, and processed foods.

Do ALA fatty acids protect your heart like EPA and DHA?

Probably, although data on ALA heart protection are not as clear as those on EPA/DHA. The Lyon Heart Study looked at patients with a history of heart attacks and randomized them to either a control diet (patients made no changes in normal eating habits) or to a Mediterranean diet that was rich in ALA-derived foods. The patients in the group with higher ALA intake had a *70 percent lower risk* of coronary events and sudden death. These results look very promising, but they may be skewed by the fact that the ALA diet group was also eating more olive oil and fish than the control group. The final answer may be hard to come by because of all the variables.

However, we do know that omega-3 fatty acids, in any form, provide you with the good fats your body needs and are especially heart-healthy when used as substitutes for saturated and trans fats.

Your Heart Goes Nuts for Nuts

There's no question that nuts are good for your heart. Research shows that eating just a handful of nuts four or five days a week can significantly lower your risk of coronary heart disease.

How does this happen? Nuts have many attributes that contribute to lowering your risk for heart disease. Most types are rich in the healthy monounsaturated fatty acid called oleic acid and low in unhealthy saturated fatty acids. In addition, nuts contain the antioxidant vitamin E and folic acid and are high in fiber. They also contain arginine, a precursor to nitric acid, which helps blood vessels to relax and helps prevent blood clotting. As I said earlier, particular nuts, including pine nuts, contain ALA, a type of omega-3 fatty acid that protects against heart disease by preventing dangerous heart arrhythmias.

Like all plant foods, nuts and peanuts (which are actually legumes and have greater amounts of protein and arginine than any nut) are cholesterol-free. Peanuts also contain resveratrol, a substance thought to contribute to the heart-healthy benefits of red wine.

Heart Smart Nutty Fact

Nuts can lower bad cholesterol levels, raise HDL levels, lower homo-cysteine levels, improve arterial health, improve arterial vasodilation, protect against clotting, and reduce the risk of arrhythmias.

The Proven Benefits of Eating Nuts

Clinical trials have consistently shown that eating nuts regularly can reduce your risk of cardiovascular disease. Large studies, such as the Adventis Health Study and the U.S. Physicians Health Study, show a direct relationship between eating nuts and protecting against heart disease. Data from the Harvard School of Public Health's Nurses Health Study showed that substituting peanuts and nuts for saturated fats or refined carbohydrates reduced the risk of heart disease by up to 45 percent.

In 2002, researchers at Harvard University's Brigham and Women's Hospital reported on the U.S. Physicians Health Study, which stated that consuming at least an ounce of nuts twice a week cut the risk of sudden cardiac death in half and lowered the risk of coronary heart disease by 30 percent!

How Many Nuts Should You Eat?

It doesn't take many nuts to be heart-healthy. In fact, it's quite easy to *overdo it* and run the risk of weight gain. Be aware that nuts, while great for your heart, are high-calorie snacks that contain up to 150 calories per handful. However, their fat and protein content make you feel full earlier than carbohydrates do, which means you can eat fewer of them and still have your hunger satisfied.

Eating an ounce of nuts (three to four tablespoons) five or more times a week will improve your diet and can reduce the risk of coronary heart disease by 25 to 30 percent.

Make Nuts a Part of Your Day

The key to making nuts a healthy part of your diet is to substitute them for other, less healthy foods you are currently eating. Nuts are a great way to turn that unhealthy midafternoon cookie into a heart-healthy snack.

You can make nuts a daily choice by

- Substituting a handful of nuts for a less beneficial afternoon snack

- Sprinkling nuts on a hearty salad for a complete meal
- Adding nuts to fish, chicken, or pasta dishes as a flavorful and healthy garnish
- Adding nuts to your breakfast yogurt or breakfast cereal
- Adding nuts to pancakes and muffins
- Eating desserts made with peanut butter or nuts

Sterols and Stanols: Plants That Lower Your Cholesterol

Who knew that just spreading some "butter" on your bread could lower your heart risk?

Sterols and stanols, substances found naturally in all plants, have a chemical structure similar to that of human cholesterol—but they actually help *lower* blood levels of cholesterol rather than add to them. They do this by blocking cholesterol absorption in the intestines. When the intestines are not able to absorb cholesterol, which is needed for normal cellular function, the liver turns on its LDL receptors and starts sweeping out the bad cholesterol from the bloodstream. This lowers your bad LDL cholesterol levels, with an average decrease of 10 percent, and reduces your risk of coronary heart disease. Sterols and stanols have little or no effect on the good cholesterol or triglycerides.

Good natural sources of stanols and sterols are nuts, grains, legumes, breads, cereals, seeds, and leaves. But these beneficial substances are also now available as a margarine-type spread and snacks (marketed as Benecol Spread and Benecol Smart Chews, respectively). Just spread some on bread or corn and watch your cholesterol level drop.

How much of these plant substances should you eat? Though the typical amount consumed is 160 to 400 mg a day, you need 2 to 3 *grams* a day to lower cholesterol levels by 10 to 20 percent. This amounts to two or three pats of the spread daily. The Food and Drug Administration advises, "Diets low in saturated fat and cholesterol that include two servings of foods that provide a daily total of at least 3.4 grams of plant stanol esters in two meals may reduce the risk of heart disease."

The Joy of Soy: It Lowers Your Cholesterol, Too

Soy products are another heart-healthy food source and help protect you from cardiovascular disease. A meta-analysis of thirty-eight clinical trials published in the *New England Journal of Medicine* by Dr. James Anderson found that people who consumed soy, rather than animal protein, significantly reduced serum concentrations of total and LDL cholesterol as well as triglyceride levels.

Soy does more than just lower your LDL cholesterol and triglyceride levels. Soy products also protect your heart by *raising good HDL levels; helping to reduce the risk of blood clotting; improving endothelial function; and preventing the oxidation of LDL cholesterol,* one of the early triggers of atherosclerosis.

Soy foods, which are low in fat and cholesterol, include soybeans, soy nuts, tempeh (chewy soybean cake), miso, tofu (soybean curd that comes in firm, soft, or silken consistencies), soy flour, and soymilk. They are excellent substitutes for products that are high in saturated fats and cholesterol. For example, you can use soymilk instead of milk, tofu instead of meat or cheese, and tempeh instead of meat.

Soy, a Wonderful Protein Alternative

Source of Soy	Protein (grams)
Soy milk	6.0
Tofu (3 oz.)	8.5
Tofu yogurt (8 oz.)	8.0
Miso (1 tbsp.)	2.0
Soybeans (½ cup)	13.0
Soy nuts (¼ cup)	12.0

The Food and Drug Administration has approved a soy product health claim that states "a diet that includes food with soy protein may lower an individual's risk of heart disease provided the diet is low in saturated fat and cholesterol." Soy products that can make this claim must contain at least 6.25 grams of soy protein, be low in fat (less than 3 grams), low in saturated fat (less than 1 gram), and low in cholesterol (less than 20 milligrams).

It is thought that 25 grams of soy protein a day (equivalent to four cups of soymilk) may help lower your cardiovascular risk. Soy protein, which is extracted from soybeans, is a complete protein that has a very healthy mixture of fats: it is low in saturated fat, contains 8 percent

---

Heart Smart Soy Fact

Twenty-five grams of soy protein per day reduce your total cholesterol levels by an average of 9 percent and your LDL cholesterol by 13 percent. This lowers your risk of heart disease by up to 20 to 30 percent, because for every 1 percent reduction in cholesterol you can expect a 2 to 3 percent reduction in the risk of coronary heart disease.

---

omega-3 fatty acids (ALA), and has 25 percent monounsaturated fatty acids.

Though soy is available as a supplement and as an extract that contain isoflavones, these forms have not yet been proven to be as effective at lowering cholesterol as soy protein foods that contain isoflavones.

Alcohol and Heart Disease: Cheers to a Healthy Heart

There are two dates in history that many wine lovers and the wine industry will celebrate forever. The first was November 17, 1991. That was the date that the TV program *60 Minutes* first aired a segment called "The French Paradox." The second date was January 8, 2003. That was when the highly respected *New England Journal of Medicine* reported a study showing that moderate alcohol consumption could save lives.

While the information that alcohol had heart-protective effects wasn't exactly new, the reports from these two well-respected sources catapulted wine and alcohol into the limelight in the war against heart disease. Let's look at what they said.

The French Paradox

Despite a diet rich in cream, cheese, meat, and butter, only about 7 percent of French adults are obese. That's incredibly low compared to 20 percent of English adults and 35 percent of Americans. The French also have a relatively sedate lifestyle and smoke plenty of cigarettes—a recipe, you would think, for a high rate of heart attacks. For some reason, though, the French don't die from cardiovascular disease as often as the rest of us.

In 1979 a study was done to compare the heart attack risk of the French and the English. The result? Even though both groups had a similar activity level, the same smoking habits, and equivalent fat intake, the French had *one-third less* risk of heart disease compared to the British.

Despite their best efforts to find any differences between the two groups, researchers could find only one: wine intake. The French drank more wine than their English counterparts. The conclusion, therefore, was that wine consumption helps protect against coronary heart disease.

Do I hear you say, "Let the drinking begin!"? I wouldn't go that far that fast. Scientists have spent the past twenty years trying to prove the heart-protective effects of wine and alcohol, so before you start building your wine cellar, let's look at all the facts.

What Do the Data Show?

For the most part, the French Paradox study has produced more questions than answers.

- Is red wine better than white wine for your heart?
- Is wine better than beer?
- Is hard liquor as protective as wine?
- How much alcohol is healthy?
- How much alcohol is too much?
- Should doctors really recommend alcohol for heart disease?
- If wine is protective, then why can't we just drink grape juice, since it contains the same protective substances?
- Are raisins just as healthful as grapes?
- Is it the skin, the juice, or the seed of the grape that is heart-protective, or is the alcohol most helpful?
- How does wine actually protect the heart?

Some of these questions can now be answered, but researchers all over the world are still working furiously to try to answer many of them. But the fact is that in more than a hundred clinical studies involving more than a quarter million people, an *inverse relationship* between moderate alcohol consumption and coronary heart disease has been shown. There is now credible and consistent evidence indicating that drinking alcohol in small to moderate amounts does have beneficial and protective cardio-vascular effects.

Two of the most publicized clinical trials evaluating the drinking of small to moderate amounts of alcohol were published in early 2003 in the most esteemed medical journals in the country. One study showed that consuming small to moderate amounts of alcohol reduces the risk of heart attacks by close to 30 percent; the other showed a reduction in the risk of strokes by a similar amount.

What Kind of Alcohol Is the Most Heart-Healthy?

The most common question I'm asked about alcohol is, "Which drink will provide me with the most heart protection?" When patients ask this question, I tell them there are studies suggesting that wine, in particular red wine, *may be* the most heart-protective alcoholic drink. It's a little bit cloudy, though, because when wine drinkers are compared to beer or hard-liquor drinkers, wine drinkers tend to lead healthier lifestyles, consume more fruits and vegetables, have a higher fiber intake, and have a lower incidence of smoking. So is it the total lifestyle or the wine that gets the credit?

In general, the data about the effects of the different types of alcohol on the heart do not support a clear winner. When dietary and lifestyle factors are corrected for in most of the clinical trials, all types of alcohol appear to have similar protective effects for the heart. In general, intake of wine, beer, or hard liquor in the moderate, recommended amounts is probably equally protective against coronary heart disease.

How Does Alcohol Protect Your Heart?

Alcohol has a number of different heart-protective properties. Its primary heart benefits are raising good HDL levels and inhibiting the clot-producing effects of platelets, which can cause heart attacks.

Heart Smart Alcohol Fact

Approximately half of the cardiovascular benefits of alcohol have been linked to the increase in HDL cholesterol.

Alcohol's Effects on HDL Cholesterol

Alcohol causes a good change in lipoproteins. By drinking one to two drinks a day, you can raise your HDL cholesterol levels up to 12 to 15 percent. This is about the same amount of increase in HDL cholesterol levels that you can expect with exercise or fibric acid medications (see chapter 14).

Alcohol and Clot Prevention

The other major heart-protective property of alcohol is its ability to "thin out the blood." Much like aspirin, alcohol inhibits prostaglandin synthesis, which decreases platelet aggregation—medical terminology that simply means platelets become less "sticky" and you are less likely to form

---

One Heart-Related Downside of Drinking Alcohol

Alcohol does appear to have heart-protective benefits. But drinking alcohol also has a negative aspect affecting the heart: its connections with triglycerides. Like all carbohydrates, alcohol increases triglyceride levels, which can be dangerous. The increase in triglycerides is especially pronounced if the drinker already has high triglyceride levels.

---

clots, the cause of heart attacks and strokes. Some research has shown that the resveratrol in red wine provides blood-thinning properties above and beyond those in alcohol, though the point is still under debate.

The French Paradox Revisited

Though many people believe that alcohol consumption accounts for the French Paradox, others don't agree. In 2003, researchers from the University of Pennsylvania concluded that alcohol wasn't keeping the French from having heart attacks, it was the smaller amounts of food they eat. Smaller portions and fewer calories, they reported, were the reasons the French could eat such rich foods yet stay slim.

The researchers reported some startling findings. They found that restaurants in America serve, on average, 25 percent larger portions when compared to restaurants in Paris. Even chain restaurants with locations in both the United States and France served larger portions in their U.S.

The Cardiovascular Benefits of Alcohol

- Alcohol raises HDL cholesterol.
- Alcohol inhibits platelet aggregation, acting as a blood thinner in the same way as aspirin.
- Wine contains flavonoids, which act as antioxidants.
- Grape skins contain antioxidants and nitrous oxide, which help dilate arteries.
- Polyphenols (found in the skins of red grapes) suppress endothelin-1, a powerful blood vessel constrictor.

---

outlets. Chinese American restaurants served meals that were a mind-boggling 72 percent larger than their French counterparts.

Still other researchers believe that there are different facts behind the French Paradox. They think that the French have less heart disease because they eat fewer processed foods, take smaller bites, take longer to eat meals, and eat larger meals at regular intervals.

Any or all of these factors, in addition to drinking red wine, are likely to play a role in the mystery of the French Paradox.

The Bottom Line

Alcohol plays a limited role in the prevention and treatment of coronary heart disease. While it has been shown that light to moderate alcohol consumption reduces the risk of coronary heart disease in middle-aged and older adults by about 20 to 30 percent when compared to non-drinkers, alcohol use should be looked at with caution, with the primary focus on diet, exercise, and risk factor modification.

I agree with the recommendations of the Adult Treatment Program III, an expert panel that makes recommendations for cholesterol treatment: "No more than two drinks a day for men and no more than one drink per day for women should be consumed," and "Persons who do not drink should not be encouraged to initiate regular alcohol consumption." I would add to those words a reminder that drinking alcohol has many potential negatives, including taking in excess calories and possibly gaining weight; elevating triglyceride levels; and, with high levels of alcohol intake, multiple adverse effects, including higher levels of death from heart disease.

Garlic and Your Heart: What's All the Stink?

In the constant search for natural foods and supplements that can help lower your risk for coronary heart disease, garlic has recently come under the spotlight. The intensely flavored bulb does appear to have some beneficial cardiovascular effects (just ask Larry King), but just how garlic delivers these benefits is still being studied

Garlic is part of the family of sulfur-containing compounds in the allium family, which also includes onions and leeks. Some research suggests that the allicin in garlic works just like the statin drugs, inhibiting the cholesterol-producing enzyme called HMG-CoA reductase. Other research suggests that garlic may have some antioxidant effects and that high doses of garlic may decrease clotting. A number of smaller-size trials suggest that garlic's cardiovascular benefits come through both cholesterol-lowering and blood-thinning.

Garlic Lowers Cholesterol

More than twenty randomized trials have shown a small decrease in total and LDL cholesterol—between 1 and 25 mg/dL—with various garlic preparations. However, no significant effect has been seen on good HDL cholesterol levels or triglycerides.

Despite all the interest, there have been no clinical trials to show any life-saving benefits for garlic, as there have been for cholesterol-lowering drugs and omega-3 fatty acids. So while it seems that garlic very mildly lowers cholesterol levels, to date there is no proof that it lowers heart attack risk or saves lives.

The bottom line is that garlic may help and probably doesn't hurt. If you enjoy garlic there is no reason to avoid it, and it may provide a modest assist in LDL cholesterol lowering. The only real side effects if you decide to increase your garlic intake may be smelly breath, body odor, abdominal pain, and gas, which are, of course, more of a nuisance for you—and your friends—than dangerous.

Vitamin E: Heart-Healthy Miracle or Heart-Healthy Flop?

Everybody wants vitamin E to be the wonder pill for cardiovascular disease protection. It just makes sense that this vitamin would help protect your heart. Coronary heart disease and atherosclerosis are caused in part by oxidation, and vitamin E acts as an antioxidant. It seems like a match made in Heaven, but it's not always that simple.

Finally, after years of debate it appears that the great vitamin E debate may be coming to a close. Though initially it looked like there was great promise, the largest and most respected clinical trials consistently have been unable to prove any significant cardiovascular protection from vitamin E. In fact, the latest trial looking at vitamin E not only showed no benefits on the heart, but there was even a suggestion that high doses of vitamin E may *worsen* or *trigger* heart failure.

What Is Vitamin E?

Vitamin E is a powerful antioxidant that is a natural part of many foods, including green leafy vegetables, fortified cereals, nuts (almonds, hazelnuts, peanuts), and vegetable oils. It is also available as a supplement in the form of alpha-tocopherol. Like other antioxidants, vitamin E was thought to protect your cells by blunting the effects of the potentially dangerous "free radicals" that are produced by a number of diseases, including cardiovascular disease.

Vitamin E and Heart Disease

Vitamin E was once thought to help prevent or delay coronary heart disease by limiting the oxidation of LDL cholesterol, a process that promotes the deposit of cholesterol plaque on the heart artery walls and triggers atherosclerosis and heart attacks. Initially, there seemed to be convincing data to support this theory. But once researchers really started looking at vitamin E in patients prospectively over a number of years, the vitamin E heart-protection theory lost favor.

Two major clinical trials debunked the vitamin E heart-protection theory. The Heart Outcomes Prevention Evaluation (HOPE) Study and a study sponsored by the National Heart, Lung, and Blood Institute (NHLBI) did not find any heart-protection benefits in patients taking vitamin E. The HOPE Study randomized ten thousand patients at high risk for heart attack and stroke to either 400 IU of vitamin E daily or a placebo and found no difference in the rate of cardiovascular events, hospitalizations, heart attack, chest pain, or death. The NHLBI study failed to show any cardiovascular benefits from taking 400 IU of vitamin E a day.

The most recent trial looking at vitamin E and the heart was a follow-up of the HOPE Study called HOPE-TOO. This new study found that patients over age fifty-five with heart disease, stroke, or diabetes plus at least one other cardiovascular risk factor who took vitamin E supplements experienced an *increased risk* of congestive heart failure.

The Bottom Line

The bottom line is that in large clinical trials, vitamin E has not been shown to have protective cardiovascular effects and currently cannot be recommended as a supplement for heart disease prevention. Instead of taking vitamin E supplements, you can do as the American Heart Association recommends (and I agree with) and "eat a diet high in food sources of antioxidants and other heart-protecting nutrients, such as fruits, vegetables, whole grains, and nuts . . . to reduce the risk of cardiovascular disease."

Fiber: A Little Goes a Long Way

If you are like most of us, your diet could probably use a real fiber boost. For some reason, when I talk to patients about fiber I often just get a blank stare as my only reply. Yes, prunes and bran muffins are good sources of fiber, but trust me, there are other really good (and better-tasting) sources of fiber.

Adding fiber to your daily diet really helps protect the heart. Study after study has shown that those countries with the highest fiber consumption also tend to have the lowest rates of coronary heart disease.

Your best bet, to get the 20 to 35 grams of fiber a day that is recommended for heart health, is to eat fiber from each of the main fiber-rich food classes throughout the day. There are a number of readily available sources of fiber: oatmeal, legumes (beans and peas), whole grains, fruits, and vegetables.

Fiber Lowers Cholesterol Levels

Your body cannot break down fiber, meaning it passes through your digestive system essentially unchanged. As fiber passes through your intestines it helps block the reabsorption of cholesterol, thereby lowering your blood cholesterol levels by 5 to 10 percent. This ability to lower cholesterol levels is the likely explanation as to why countries with the highest fiber intakes also seem to have the lowest rates of coronary heart disease.

I try hard to push my patients to increase their fiber intake. I have seen that by focusing on adding plant-based, high-fiber foods into your diet, you almost by default end up eating less calorie-rich, fat-laden animal foods—making it a win-win situation.

A Cardiologist's Take on the Atkins, South Beach, and Mediterranean Diets

Everyone wants a quick fix when it comes to losing weight. Though it may have taken you five or even ten years to put on the extra weight you're carrying, you want it all to come off in just eight weeks.

The quick-fix approach to heart health and weight loss all but guarantees disappointment and failure. While quick-fix diets do deliver quick results, they simply don't work for the long term, and can even be dangerous in the short term.

Since I'm always asked my opinion on some of the current popular diets, the following section includes my take on three of the most popular: the Atkins Diet, the South Beach Diet, and the Mediterranean Diet. As you read, keep in mind that any diet is simply a short-term plan to lose weight. To be heart-healthy you need to forget about going on a diet and instead start living a heart-healthy lifestyle.

The Atkins Diet   Dr. Robert C. Atkins introduced his approach to weight loss and dieting in his book *Dr. Atkins' Diet Revolution* way back in 1972. His controversial ideas exploded in popularity in the late 1990s and led to a craze of dieting, a billion-dollar-a-year Atkins industry, and a stunned and confused medical community.

Dr. Atkins' philosophy is that overweight and obesity are caused by a "disturbed carbohydrate imbalance" rather than by overeating. He claimed that by following his low-carbohydrate, high-protein diet, people would lose weight by eating calorie- and fat-laden "bacon and eggs for breakfast, heavy cream in their coffee, mayonnaise in their salads, butter sauce on their lobster, spareribs, roast duck, pastrami, and cheesecake."

To the surprise of many experts, many people on the Atkins Diet did lose weight, and they also, according to Dr. Atkins, "gained energy, cheerfulness, and self-confidence."

The Atkins philosophy is built around the metabolism of carbohydrates. Carbohydrates (which include grains, pastas, fruits, and potatoes, which account for about 50 percent of the calories the typical American consumes in a day) are organic compounds that include sugars, starches, and celluloses. When carbohydrates are metabolized, they serve as major sources of energy in our diet. Dr. Atkins believed that if you avoid carbohydrates your body will switch from burning carbohydrates to burning fats.

The most controversial part of the original Atkins plan is that followers were told to eat a high intake of animal fat and protein and to avoid sugars and carbohydrates.

The American Heart Association and most cardiologists, including myself, do not support high-animal-fat, high-protein diets such as the Atkins Diet. This is because they have not been proven effective for long-term weight loss; restrict many healthy foods, including fruit; and likely *increase* the risk of many diseases, including cardiovascular disease.

Of the dozens of patients I have seen take on the Atkins diets, 100 percent who lost weight with the Atkins Diet regained most or all of it within a year. Even more disturbing, a number of young people I encountered who followed the Atkins Diet developed severe heart artery blockages shortly after starting it.

The South Beach Diet   Written by cardiologist Arthur Agatston, *The South Beach Diet: The Delicious Doctor-Designed, Foolproof Plan for Fast and Healthy Weight Loss* made an immediate splash when it hit bookstores in 2003. The South Beach Diet, like the Atkins Diet, is based on a low-carbohydrate eating plan. The biggest difference is that the South Beach Diet promotes a more sensible approach to protein.

Dr. Agatston's diet is based on the glycemic index of foods. Foods that contain carbohydrates cause a rapid rise in blood sugar levels, which causes a rapid rise in insulin levels. High insulin levels then immediately push blood sugar into storage, causing a rapid fall in blood sugar levels. Low blood sugar levels make you feel hungry and cause you to crave more carbohydrates to increase your blood sugar levels again. Because of this, according to Dr. Agatston, foods that cause the fastest rise and drop, putting them at the top of the glycemic index list, should be avoided; this includes refined grains (found in many white breads), potatoes, sodas, and fruit juices. Foods that are low on the glycemic index, and don't result in immediate cravings, should be a major part of your diet; these include vegetables, legumes, and fruit.

The South Beach Diet consists of three phases: an induction phase designed to "banish the craving" for carbohydrates, during which only foods containing fats and those at the lowest end of the glycemic index are allowed; a middle phase that reintroduces some carbohydrates into your diet, such as whole grains and fruits; and a maintenance phase that you stay on for the long term.

While there have been no long-term studies to assess the effects of the South Beach Diet on cholesterol levels, weight loss, or cardiovascular disease, in general I believe the diet is a reasonable approach to weight loss, particularly compared to the Atkins Diet. The South Beach Diet promotes eating healthy carbohydrates and the good fats. I do, however, recommend that you eat a more well-balanced diet, and I emphasize using exercise as the primary way to lose weight.

The Mediterranean Diet   Researchers have found that people who live in the countries that border the Mediterranean Sea (think Greece, among others) have lower levels of cholesterol, lower rates of coronary heart disease, and are less likely to die from heart attacks when compared to other civilized countries. Despite eating excess fat, people who follow the "Mediterranean Diet" have excellent heart health.

The Mediterranean Diet follows all of my rules for a Heart Smart eating plan. It is a *balanced* diet consisting mostly of grains, fruits, beans, nuts, and seeds. There is little red meat in this diet, so the saturated fat intake is very low. The fats that are consumed are polyunsaturated fats from fish and nuts and monounsaturated fats from olive oil, which raise good HDL cholesterol levels and lower bad LDL cholesterol levels.

This heart-healthy intake of good fats is one of the major reasons the Mediterranean Diet is good for you. Another reason is also attributed to the small to moderate intake of wine it includes, which is part of the way of life in this region of the world. In general the diet is a commonsense, heart-healthy, and tasty approach to eating that is easily sustainable for the long term.

However, there are two things to be careful about if you decide to go on the Mediterranean Diet: not eating too much fat, even the good kind, and not drinking too much alcohol. As I've said previously, even good fats have their potential drawbacks: they are high in calories and if eaten in excess will promote weight gain and obesity. Alcohol also has a significant set of potential negative effects, not the least of which is that it is high in calories.

Summing It Up

There are specific heart-healthy foods that can lower your risk of cardiovascular disease, heart attacks, and sudden cardiac death. Fish, nuts, soy, stanols/sterols, fiber, garlic, and moderate alcohol intake all cut your risk, while vitamin E supplements are not helpful at lowering your risk (and may even be harmful at higher doses).

Ultimately, the best approach to living a Heart Smart life is a long-term eating plan that you enjoy and that is well balanced. You can draw from both the South Beach Diet, which focuses on minimizing the simple carbohydrates and increasing healthy fat intake, and the Mediterranean Diet, which emphasizes eating fish, vegetables, nuts, whole grains, and the good fats, but the American Heart Association, the American Medical Association, the U.S. Department of Agriculture (USDA), and the Centers for Disease Control (CDC) all support a simple, well-balanced diet that is low in trans and saturated fats.

The bottom line is that if you lower your intake of bad fats and unhealthy carbohydrates and increase your amount of exercise—you burn more calories than you eat—you will lose weight and stay heart-healthy.

No one diet is best for everyone. But by understanding the principles behind a heart-healthy diet, eating foods you enjoy that fit the heart-healthy profile, and exercising, you will begin to lower your risk of heart attacks and coronary heart disease.

Chapter 14

Aspirin and Cholesterol-Lowering Drugs

Heart Medications to Save Your Life

The right heart medications lower your risk of coronary heart disease and sudden cardiac death by an average of 30 percent. You owe it to yourself to find out what these medications are and whether you should be taking them.

But, first, a word of caution: don't lose sight of the forest for the trees. The constant bombardment of mass direct-to-consumer advertising and the Internet's mountain of information about cardiovascular drugs, vitamins, herbs, and supplements can expose you to unnecessary risks and drag you down unsafe treatment paths.

As you consider heart medications, remember to keep it simple. And rather than taking a handful of unproven, unregulated, and potentially unsafe herbs and supplements each day, stick to medications that are *safe and proven* to lower your risk of heart disease and help prevent cardiovascular death.

Aspirin and cholesterol-lowering drugs are two of the primary medications used to fight coronary heart disease. In this chapter you'll learn how this dynamic duo dramatically reduces your risk of heart attacks and death by hitting heart disease right where it hurts the most—in the cholesterol plaque.

Aspirin: The Protective Wonder Drug

Aspirin, or acetylsalicylic acid, is a unique medication in our fight against coronary heart disease; it comes from salicylates, which originate from the bark of the willow tree. Aspirin is known as a "wonder drug" because it is an over-the-counter medication, inexpensive, safe (though not without potential side effects), and effective in both the prevention and treatment of coronary heart disease and stroke. The drug has been around for more than a century, primarily used for its pain-relieving effects, but for the past thirty years it also has been recognized for its cardiovascular protective effects.

Aspirin is part of a class of medications called nonsteroidal anti-inflammatory drugs, or NSAIDs. While some of the NSAIDs have caused a recent scare and may be linked to possibly causing heart attacks, aspirin has been shown to have only beneficial effects. Aspirin has been proven effective for both preventing the development of coronary heart disease and keeping it from progressing.

Heart Smart Aspirin Fact

Aspirin's effects vary depending on the dose. At a low dose aspirin has cardiovascular protective effects; at a medium dose it also provides pain-killing effects; and at a high dose it also has anti-inflammatory effects.

How Does Aspirin Protect Your Heart?

One of the last phases of atherosclerosis, the complex process that ultimately leads to heart attacks, is clotting. Under normal conditions, platelets, which circulate in the blood and are designed to be protective, are "slippery": they slip and slide through the blood without attaching to anything. In response to trauma, such as a cut or a scrape, platelets activate and change from slippery to "sticky." Sticky platelets clog up cuts and scrapes to help prevent excessive bleeding. They are your body's form of a Band-Aid.

Unfortunately, platelets also react to atherosclerotic plaque growing inside your heart arteries. As platelets encounter this cholesterol plaque they recognize that something is wrong and "activate," changing from slippery to sticky. The sticky platelets then form a clot and attract other clotting factors to the area. Your platelets think they are helping to repair your damaged arteries, but in fact they are only making the situation worse, and setting you up for a heart attack.

Aspirin prevents clots. It works its magic right on atherosclerotic plaque, the heart and soul of coronary heart disease.

Aspirin works by keeping your platelets slippery. Slippery platelets can't form clots, and without clots, heart attacks don't occur. If you want to get technical about it, aspirin inhibits an enzyme called cyclooxygenase. By inhibiting this enzyme, aspirin decreases the output of a major platelet-clotting factor called thromboxane A2. Lower levels of thromboxane A2 reduce your risk of clotting and lower your heart attack risk.

Aspirin's Side Effects and Risks

Aspirin has both potentially dangerous side effects and merely bothersome side effects. The obvious and *most dangerous side effect* of a drug that inhibits clot formation is bleeding. Aspirin may promote bleeding as well as limit your ability to stop bleeding from any sort of trauma.

The two major bleeding problems that can result from taking aspirin are gastrointestinal bleeding and bleeding strokes. The risk of major bleeding is relatively small, but if it occurs, it can be life-threatening. For every thousand patients treated with aspirin, none to two will have bleeding strokes, and two to four will have major gastrointestinal bleeding episodes.

The *most common bothersome side effects* from aspirin are stomach irritation and upset. Aspirin can irritate the lining of the stomach, causing some discomfort or even ulcers with extended use. The gastrointestinal side effects of aspirin can be reduced or minimized by using an enteric-coated aspirin product.

Is Aspirin Right for You?

Aspirin may be right for you whether you are trying to prevent coronary heart disease (primary prevention) or are trying to keep the disease from progressing (secondary prevention).

However, always weigh the risks and benefits of aspirin and talk to your doctor about whether aspirin is safe for you to use.

Primary Prevention

Taking aspirin for the primary prevention of coronary heart disease is not for everyone, but most adults should at least consider it. If you have no history of bleeding problems and no allergies to aspirin, I generally recommend a daily low dose of aspirin for men over age forty-five and for women over age fifty-five. Recently published data show that older women can reduce their risk of heart attack and stroke with low-dose aspirin. Those who have multiple cardiac risk factors or diabetes can start taking aspirin at a younger age.

When the U.S. Preventive Services Task Force, a federal agency that writes guidelines for health care professionals, reviewed the multiple, major primary-prevention clinical trials involving aspirin, the members concluded that overall *aspirin produced a significant, nearly 30 percent reduction in the risk of dying from heart disease or from having a first heart attack.*

Secondary Prevention

If you already have coronary heart disease, your goal is to prevent any further problems, such as heart attacks, angioplasties, bypass surgery, or sudden cardiac death. This type of prevention is called secondary prevention.

Aspirin lowers the risk of secondary heart attacks, procedures, and cardiac death by a third for all patients with coronary heart disease. Daily low-dose aspirin is highly recommended if you have any form of atherosclerosis and no history of aspirin allergies or bleeding. Don't forget that you also should take an aspirin if you think you're having a heart attack; doing so lowers your risk of dying by more than 20 percent.

What's the Right Aspirin Dosage?

The protective cardiovascular effects aspirin provides come at lower doses. From 81 mg to 325 mg is all that is needed to irreversibly damage platelets enough to prevent clotting and heart attacks. Aspirin doses above this amount only increase your bleeding risks with no proven additional heart-protective benefits.

At some point in the future, patients may be tested to determine their individual optimal aspirin dose; new research has shown that some people are resistant to the effects of aspirin. For now, though, the "one size fits all" approach to aspirin therapy is best.

The Bottom Line

Clot formation and rupture at the site of cholesterol plaque are the final steps to having a heart attack. Aspirin works by preventing clots through its action on your platelets; it prevents them from becoming sticky and keeps them slippery and promoting brisk blood flow, lowering your cardiovascular risk.

Aspirin is one of the most important medications you can use to prevent heart attacks and reduce your risk of sudden cardiac death. It is highly effective for both primary and secondary coronary heart disease prevention. If you are a man over age forty-five or a women over age fifty-five, ask your doctor if you would benefit from a low-dose daily aspirin. If you have diabetes or multiple cardiac risk factors, you may benefit from aspirin at a younger age.

As with all medications, the risks and benefits of aspirin must be considered and discussed with your doctor before you start to take it.

Taking Medication for High Cholesterol

At this point in the Heart Smart program, you know to a certainty that cholesterol plays a central role in the development of coronary heart disease. High LDL cholesterol, low HDL cholesterol, and high triglyceride levels all contribute to atherosclerosis. However, LDL cholesterol remains the *primary target* for the prevention and treatment of coronary heart disease.

Fortunately, several new medications, including new statins, new cholesterol blockers, and new combination drugs, have made treating cholesterol and atherosclerosis safer and more effective than ever. While exercise, weight loss, smoking cessation, and a heart-healthy diet should be part of every cholesterol treatment program, if your doctor decides you need medication, you can feel confident that there are many proven drugs you can take.

The Benefits of Cholesterol-Lowering Drugs

1. Keeps the endothelium happy and healthy.
2. Prevents any new atherosclerotic plaques from developing.
3. Stops the progression of existent plaques.
4. Stabilizes the fibrous cap to prevent plaque rupture (heart attacks).
5. May reduce the size and severity of existing plaques.

It's Not Just about the Numbers

If you need to bring down your cholesterol, it's time for you to start thinking differently about treatment. The old mind-set of lowering cholesterol is hindering our ability to treat and prevent heart disease. You don't want to just lower your cholesterol "numbers." Stopping or reversing atherosclerosis is the reason you want to treat your cholesterol. So don't just think about lowering your cholesterol. Instead, think about prevention, stabilization, and regression.

To stop the progression of coronary heart disease, you need to keep your LDL cholesterol level at less than 100 mg/dL. At this level you are very unlikely to develop any new cholesterol plaque. If your goal is to reverse your heart disease, you need to lower your LDL cholesterol level to less than 70 mg/dL. Taking cholesterol medications can help you do both of these things.

Heart Smart Plaque Fact

Plaque stabilization and *plaque regression* are the primary goals in treating coronary heart disease. A stable plaque with a 60 percent artery blockage will rarely hurt you. An unstable plaque, however, with a 35 percent blockage, can rupture, causing a heart attack or death.

Balancing the Risk of Drugs

Like all medications, the cholesterol-lowering medications have some side effects. The question you should ask yourself and your doctor is, "Do the benefits of the medication outweigh its risks?"

To help make the decision, and to avoid the small but real risks associated with cholesterol medications:

- Inform your doctor of all other medications you use.
- Take liver function blood tests at least every four months while taking cholesterol medications.
- Watch for new symptoms, including muscle aches, joint aches, nausea, vomiting, abdominal pain, or brown-colored urine.
- Talk to your doctor immediately if you have questions or concerns or to learn about potential side effects.

The Cholesterol Drugs: From A(dvicor) to Z(etia)

Cholesterol medications are broken down into five different classes based on their cholesterol-lowering mechanism: *statins*, *bile acid resins*, *niacin*, *fibrates*, and *cholesterol absorption inhibitors*. There are also two new "combination" drugs that provide a little extra punch by providing one drug from each of two different classes in one tablet.

Each class of cholesterol medication has its own special niche. Fibrates, for example, are known for lowering triglycerides, while niacin is the best drug for raising good cholesterol. Statins are the best drugs for lowering bad LDL cholesterol. The medication you take should be targeted to your particular needs—what might be right for your wife or best friend may be the completely wrong drug for you.

The following section explains the risks and benefits of each drug class as well as how each is used. I start with the most prescribed drugs in the world, the statins.

Statins: The Plaque Stabilizers

As the saying goes, the proof of the pudding is in the eating, and as far as statins go, the proof is in the clinical trials. There has been no shortage of well-constructed, highly scrutinized, national and international trials on statin benefits by top doctors, research hospitals, and government research centers, and all have proven that statins provide overwhelmingly positive cardiovascular effects.

Statins are prescribed to lower cholesterol, protect you from the damage of coronary heart disease, and prevent heart attacks. They decrease your risk of dying if you have coronary heart disease with either high cholesterol or normal cholesterol or if you have a history of heart failure, heart attack, angioplasty, or bypass surgery. Each year the number of prescriptions for these drugs grows, yet only a small fraction of patients who could benefit from statins are actually taking them at present. Everyone with documented coronary heart disease or at high risk for the disease can lower their risk of dying by taking a statin drug.

Statins are some of the most important drugs to emerge in the past twenty years. Also known as HMG-CoA reductase inhibitors, they lower cholesterol by blocking HMG-CoA reductase, an enzyme that controls the rate of cholesterol production in the liver. By blocking this enzyme, statins lower cholesterol in two ways:

1. Slowing down the production of cholesterol in the liver

2. Increasing the liver's ability to remove bad cholesterol from the blood

Statins provide a powerful and consistent drop in total cholesterol and LDL cholesterol, routinely resulting in reductions of up to 60 percent. They also effectively lower triglyceride levels. Statins are truly workhorses when it comes to lowering LDL cholesterol and are usually chosen as first-line therapy to treat and reverse coronary heart disease.

Besides Lowering Cholesterol, What Else Do Statins Do?

In addition to their amazing cholesterol-lowering capability, statins have many other beneficial qualities. In fact, many of their most important and effective properties appear to be those outside cholesterol-lowering. Statins can reduce the occurrences of cardiovascular events, myocardial infarction, and death by

- Improving endothelial function
- Regressing the lipid core
- Stabilizing the fibrous atherosclerotic plaque
- Decreasing atherosclerotic inflammation
- Decreasing clot formation
- Promoting vasodilation

New research has also shown that statins may even positively affect conditions outside the cardiovascular system, including diabetes, macular degeneration, osteoporosis, and Alzheimer's disease.

The Nuts and Bolts of Statins

Currently there are six statin drugs on the U.S. market. They are atorvastatin (Lipitor), fluvastatin (Lescol), lovastatin (Mevacor), pravastatin (Pravachol), rosuvastatin (Crestor), and simvastatin (Zocor). All have a sustained effect and are taken once daily. Since your liver makes more cholesterol during the night than the day, there is an advantage to taking the medicine at night, when it can block the most cholesterol from being produced.

Statins begin lowering cholesterol levels in just a few weeks, with the maximum effect seen in four to eight weeks. Once you have been on the medicine for about eight to twelve weeks, your doctor will likely check to see how your cholesterol levels are responding. While you're taking the drug, you should also have regular liver function blood tests to ensure that the statin is not causing liver inflammation as an unwanted side effect.

Statins and Their Dosage

Generic Name	Brand Name	Dosage (mg)
Atorvastatin	Lipitor	10, 20, 40, 80
Fluvastatin	Lescol	20, 40
Lovastatin	Mevacor	10, 20, 40
Pravastatin	Pravachol	10, 20, 40
Rosuvastatin	Crestor	5, 10, 20
Simvastatin	Zocor	5, 10, 20, 40, 80

Statins' Side Effects

Statins' disadvantages are relatively small. Most are minor, irritating side effects, including stomach upset, gas, belching, constipation, and abdominal cramps. Achy, tender muscles are also fairly common, but these conditions often improve as your body adjusts to the medication over time.

Two side effects of statins, however, though uncommon, can be potentially dangerous.

The first is called rhabdomyolysis. Rhabdomyolysis is a particularly worrisome concern because if it's left undiagnosed it can be fatal. Rhabdomyolysis is a breakdown of muscle in the body. When muscles break down, they flood the bloodstream and eventually overwhelm the kidneys, causing them to shut down and fail.

While taking a statin, be vigilant in looking for the warning signs of rhabdomyolysis. Symptoms include muscle pains, muscle cramping, and brown/cloudy urine. If you develop any of these symptoms, notify your doctor immediately. Rhabdomyolysis can be detected with a simple muscle enzyme blood test called a creatine kinase.

The second potentially dangerous side effect of statins is liver toxicity. Keeping close track of liver function through blood tests while you take a statin will minimize this problem. Make sure that you have regular blood tests, at least every four months, to check for early liver inflammation. The good news is that if your liver is affected by a statin, function almost always returns to normal once you stop taking the drug

Both liver toxicity and rhabdomyolysis are more common when different classes of cholesterol drugs are used in combination.

Bile Acid Resins: Cholesterol-Lowering Drugs

The bile acid resins (often simply called "resins") are another option for reducing LDL cholesterol. Resins have been around for years, but the success of statins has caused their use to dramatically decline. The bile acid resins are now used primarily to lower cholesterol only when all else fails.

How Do Resins Lower Cholesterol?

Bile, an important digestive enzyme, is made by bile acids in the liver with the help of cholesterol. The resins work by blocking bile acids from recycling in the intestines, forcing the liver to remove more cholesterol from the blood to make more bile. When the liver cranks up its need for cholesterol, less of the substance is left in the bloodstream to cause damage inside your arteries. The resins' working mechanism isn't high-tech, but it is fairly effective.

Used alone, bile acids produce a modest 10 to 20 percent decrease in LDL cholesterol. They are more effective when used in combination with other types of cholesterol-lowering drugs such as the statins.

The Nuts and Bolts of Bile Acid Resins

Two main bile acid resins are currently available in the United States: cholestyramine and colestipol (Colestid). A third drug, colesevelam (Wel-Chol), technically is not a bile acid resin, but it has similar actions and usually is grouped with the resins as a cholesterol-lowering drug. The bile acid resins can be taken as a tablet, in powder form, or as a chewable bar.

All three resin drugs are generally considered safe because the body does not absorb them. However, because they work by binding to bile acids in the intestines, they have a tendency to cause a number of side effects and to interfere with a number of other medications you may also be taking. If you do take other medications, be sure to take them at least four to six hours after or one hour before you take the resin. Be aware that there are interactions between resins and coumadin (and other anticoagulants), antibiotics, thyroid medications, diuretics, and grapefruit juice.

Bile Acid Resin Side Effects

The most common of the many potential side effects of resins are gastrointestinal-related and include constipation, diarrhea, stomach irritation, abdominal pain, nausea, vomiting, gas, belching, abdominal bloating, and heartburn. The drugs should be used carefully or not at all if you have severe constipation, gallstones, high triglyceride levels, vitamin deficiencies, major gastrointestinal disorders, severe obesity, bleeding disorders, or thyroid disorders. You also need to be aware that resins can actually *raise* triglyceride levels while being only mildly effective in elevating good HDL cholesterol.

As you should do while taking any of the cholesterol-lowering drugs, be sure to have liver function tests every three to four months and to have routine blood tests to check your cholesterol and triglyceride levels.

Niacin (Nicotinic Acid): Medication to Raise Your Good Cholesterol

Niacin is to HDL cholesterol as statins are to LDL cholesterol. Niacin has positive effects on all the lipids but is the first drug of choice if you have low HDL cholesterol levels.

Because high good-cholesterol levels are very protective against the atherosclerotic process—so much so that it is rare for people with high HDL levels to have heart attacks—you want your level to be as high as it can be. Diet and lifestyle changes are important parts of HDL treatment, but many times medical therapy is needed to produce a big enough change.

That's where niacin comes in.

- Niacin elevates HDL cholesterol.
- Niacin lowers triglycerides.
- Niacin lowers LDL cholesterol.

Niacin also is the only current drug that can treat some emerging cardiac risk factors (for more on emerging risk factors, see chapter 7). It lowers lipoprotein (a) and raises a subfraction of HDL called apo A-1—a powerful protector against atherosclerosis.

What Is Niacin?

Niacin is a natural form of vitamin B_3 that's found in dairy products, eggs, and meat. It is also available in pill form over the counter; however, higher doses are needed to significantly affect cholesterol levels. Prescription-strength niacin is required to provide doses that are high enough to affect your cholesterol while causing fewer side effects. There are a number of ever-changing theories on how niacin works, but we don't quite have our finger on it yet.

Flush Away Niacin's Side Effects

The side effects niacin can produce can be quite scary if you are not prepared. The most common side effect is called flushing (or hot flashes), which causes warmth, redness, itching, or tingling, usually on the face and head. However, you can minimize flushing and niacin's other possible side effects, such as dizziness, headache, gas, nausea, and diarrhea, if you take the right steps.

To minimize niacin's side effects, do the following:

- Take before bedtime.
- Take an aspirin or NSAID (such as ibuprofen) half an hour before.
- Take with a low-fat snack.
- Start at a low dose and gradually increase it over weeks to months.
- Take the sustained, slow-release form.
- Avoid alcohol, hot drinks, and spicy foods.
- Take the niacin tablet whole, not crushed, broken, or chewed.
- Give it time; your body tends to get accustomed to most side effects.

Flushing is so common that the pharmaceutical companies that make niacin products provide educational booklets, guidelines, and even 1-800 hotlines to help you deal with the side effects and to answer your concerns. If your doctor prescribes a niacin product for you to take for your cholesterol, always ask for samples and the educational pamphlet.

One of the key ways to minimize side effects is to start taking niacin at a low dose and then titrate up slowly. Generally the beginning dosage is 500 mg once each evening; this is increased by 500 mg every month until the maximum dosage of 2,000 mg a day is reached. Unfortunately, it usually takes the maximum dose to raise HDL or lower Lp(a) to the desired levels. If side effects occur, you may need to slow down the titration schedule, which, of course, will make it longer until you reach the maximum dosage.

Niacin should be used with caution if you have liver problems, diabetes, or gout, or if you use alcohol heavily.

Fibrates (Fibric Acid Derivatives): Triglyceride-Lowering Drugs

All cholesterol-lowering drugs "specialize" in affecting one particular type of cholesterol or fat. For example, the statins work best at lowering

LDL cholesterol; niacin specializes in raising the good HDL cholesterol. Fibrates are good all-around cholesterol medications, but their most powerful niche is in lowering triglyceride levels.

Triglycerides are a form of fat found in food and body fat, and they are also carried in the blood as part of the cholesterol particle. Your body stores the extra calories you eat as triglycerides, which are stored in fat cells. An elevated level of triglycerides is called hypertriglyceridemia and is associated with atherosclerosis. Triglyceride levels are checked as part of the screening cholesterol panel.

Because triglycerides are an independent risk factor for heart disease, even if the rest of your cholesterol numbers are in the normal range, a high triglyceride level elevates your risk of the disease.

If you have elevated triglyceride levels, fibrates are the drug treatment of choice. If you have a combination of high triglycerides and low good HDL cholesterol, fibrates also are good drugs to take.

- Fibrates lower triglycerides by 25 to 50 percent.
- Fibrates raise HDL cholesterol by 5 to 15 percent.
- Fibrates have little effect on LDL cholesterol.

Fibrate Side Effects

Many side effects are possible when you take fibrates. The most common are gastrointestinal-related and include abdominal pain, muscle aches and pain, gas, and belching. As with the statins, the fibrates also can cause a potentially life-threatening side effect called rhabdomyolysis, but its occurrence is rare. The risk of this side effect increases when a fibrate is taken in combination with other cholesterol-lowering drugs, especially a statin.

Rhabdomyolysis is a condition in which muscle begins to break down, releasing its contents into the bloodstream. If left unchecked, these breakdown products accumulate in the body and lead to kidney failure and death. Patients taking a fibrate (with or without a statin) should watch for the signs and symptoms of rhabdomyolysis: muscle cramps or pain, dark urine, nausea, vomiting, and fatigue.

Patients who have liver disease or gallbladder disease should also be sure to use fibrates with caution. Fibrates also can interact with other drugs such as coumadin and the other cholesterol-lowering medications.

Unlike the other classes of drugs that are used for cholesterol-related disorders, the fibrates have not been shown to reduce overall mortality.

Cholesterol Absorption Inhibitors:
New Drugs That Lower LDL

Cholesterol comes from two sources: your liver and your diet. The cholesterol absorption inhibitors inhibit the absorption of dietary cholesterol in the small intestine, causing the liver to feel depleted of cholesterol and therefore to increase its clearance of bad cholesterol from the bloodstream.

While there is only one drug, ezetimibe (Zetia), in the cholesterol absorption inhibitors class, the class is the first new category of cholesterol-lowering medications to come along in years. Its ability to lower cholesterol has been proven, but to date there have been no trials that show that ezetimibe has any effect on cardiovascular morbidity or mortality. Ezetimibe comes only in a 10-mg dose. It is taken once a day with or without food.

Used alone, ezetimibe lowers cholesterol only very mildly and has little or no effect on HDL cholesterol or triglycerides. It is most powerful when used in combination with a statin drug; in fact, ezetimibe's LDL-lowering capability is supercharged when it is taken this way. The combination of the two drugs blocks both of the pathways through which cholesterol enters the bloodstream, providing "dual inhibition" of cholesterol. When ezetimibe and a statin are taken together you can expect to see an additional lowering of LDL cholesterol by 10 to 30 percent, lowering of triglycerides by an additional 5 to 11 percent, and elevating of HDL cholesterol by an additional 2 to 3 percent.

Ezetimibe's Side Effects

The side effects of ezetimibe are minimal and include abdominal pain, diarrhea, dizziness, headache, and muscle aches. The drug is also safe to use with statins because it does not pose a risk to the liver.

Combination Cholesterol Medications

Treating cholesterol with medications is challenging for a number of reasons:

1. Most patients have a mixture of cholesterol issues to deal with (e.g., high LDL cholesterol and low HDL cholesterol).

2. Most cholesterol medications work only on one part of the cholesterol issue (e.g., statins lower LDL, niacin raises HDL, and fibrates lower triglycerides).

3. It's hard for patients to reach their cholesterol goals taking only one medication.

4. Patients don't like to take a lot of pills.

With these issues in mind, the pharmaceutical companies have begun making "combination" cholesterol medications, including two drugs in one tablet. So far these combination tablets have been a success with doctors because they improve cholesterol control and compliance. They also have been a success with patients by limiting the number of pills they need to take each day and by lowering costs.

The two most effective combination drugs are Advicor and Vytorin.

Advicor (Niacin + Lovastatin)

Keeping good HDL cholesterol high and bad LDL cholesterol low are critical for preventing cardiovascular disease, myocardial infarction, and death. Advicor is the only available prescription medicine that combines the LDL-lowering effects of a statin (lovastatin) with the HDL-raising effects of extended-release niacin.

- Advicor reduces LDL cholesterol by 30 to 42 percent.
- Advicor increases HDL cholesterol by 20 to 30 percent.
- Advicor reduces triglycerides by 32 to 44 percent.

The side effects, drug interactions, and other concerns associated with Advicor are the same as for the individual statin and niacin.

Vytorin (Ezetimibe + Simvastatin)

The statins are the first line of therapy for lowering LDL cholesterol. They work by blocking the production of cholesterol in the liver. For many people, however, the side effects that result from the higher doses of a statin limit its benefits, or the statin simply doesn't lower cholesterol levels enough.

When either of these situations occurs, a second cholesterol-lowering drug is added to the statin to minimize side effects while still lowering LDL cholesterol to goal. By adding the cholesterol absorption inhibitor ezetimibe (Zetia) (see above), LDL cholesterol is lowered an additional 15 to 30 precent. The "supercharged" combination of the statin simvastatin and ezetimibe causes an amazing 50 percent reduction in LDL cholesterol levels at just the starting dose.

The side effects, drug interactions, and other concerns associated with Vytorin are the same as for the individual statin and the cholesterol absorption class of drugs.

Summing It Up

Coronary artery disease and heart attacks can be characterized in three words: cholesterol, inflammation, clots. When dietary factors and lifestyle are not enough, don't hesitate to use medications to keep your risk in check.

While all of the medications I've mentioned are often used in combination to bring your cholesterol levels down to goal, always be mindful of the risks associated with these drugs and work closely with your doctor for close monitoring while taking them.

Conclusion

No More Excuses, Live Heart Smart

How badly do you want to be around to watch your children finish school and become adults? Do you want take an active part in your grandkids' lives? How do you want to spend your retirement years?

If you're not careful, work, stress, and an unhealthy lifestyle will sneak up on you and rob you of your future. In today's fast-paced world, we too often forget what is important in life. I see it all too often: one day your nose is to the grindstone working sixty to eighty hours a week, the next day it's all over. Heart attacks have no mercy on those who are "too busy" to find out their cardiac risk.

Unfortunately, my dad is a classic example. He was a workaholic who had his first heart attack and open-heart bypass surgery when he was just thirty-five years old. As he climbed his way up the corporate ladder he had his second heart attack and bypass operation ten years later. Finally, tragically, he died prematurely at age fifty-five during yet another bypass surgery, just as he was starting to think about retirement. Dad never got to meet his three beautiful granddaughters, and hardly a day goes by without me thinking how close they would be to him if he were alive today.

My dad's losing battle with heart disease is a big reason why I have dedicated my life to heart disease education and prevention. I will do whatever it takes to get the word out: *heart disease is preventable.*

Right now, in this day and age, there is no excuse for you to have a heart attack!

We may never be able to stop every single heart attack and sudden cardiac death, but we sure can come close to it. There are no mysteries here. We know what causes coronary heart disease, we know how to test for the traditional and emerging risk factors that cause it, and new technology allows us to easily detect and quantify coronary heart disease

249

earlier than ever before. Not only that, but once we find clogging of heart arteries, we have the keys to stopping it—and even reversing it—before it can do any harm.

So what's the problem? The problem lies with both patients and doctors. Doctors fail because they are not aggressive enough at screening for or treating heart disease risk factors. Patients fail because they are not aggressive enough at taking responsibility for their own health.

You will take a big step in grabbing responsibility for your heart health by following the Heart Smart 5-Step plan. This is the heart-healthy plan you have been waiting for, providing you with all the tools and information you need to empower you in your quest to beat heart disease. Use this sensible, proven, and comprehensive plan as a reference when working with your doctor to help *identify* and *minimize* your cardiac risk. You will never know your risk for a heart attack unless you take the time to test for it. Don't let a heart attack be your first sign of trouble—take action now.

I promise you won't regret it.

Index

NOTE: *Italicized* page numbers indicate illustrations.

251